Advance Praise for *Unbreakable Bonds*

We have a sacred responsibility to our military families—the Americans who on't don the uniform, but bear the burden of war and its aftermath along- de those that do. Many of us may never know the extent of their sacrifices, ut this portrait welcomes readers into the lives of caregivers—hidden eroes like Paulette Mason—at Walter Reed. Even as we can never fully repay ur military families for their service here at home, the ten mothers featured 1 this moving book give us yet another gift—their stories, courage, and nduring love. Readers of this timely portrait cannot help but feel immensely rateful and inspired."

—*Nancy Pelosi*

Movingly relates the untold story of selfless devotion, duty, and strength emonstrated by military family caregivers that is so instrumental to the ecovery and rehabilitation of our nation's wounded warriors. This is a must- ead for Americans in every corner of the country to truly understand the hallenges of postwar recovery on the home front."

—*Senator Elizabeth Dole*

The mothers of the wounded have played an important role in their recov- ry since man invented war—stories that have gone untold. Guerin and Fer- s capture the sadness and joy, compassion, persistence, fierce advocacy, and ourage in ten inspiring stories—stories of love."

—*David S. Ferriero, Archivist of the United States*

When a service member is wounded, the whole family is wounded and must e a part of the recovery. *Unbreakable Bonds* will inspire you with the never- nding commitment, strength, and love between these amazing moms and eir kids."

—*Jim Knotts, CEO of Operation Homefront*

Chronicles an amazing fusion of moral courage and limitless love. It tells e story of motherhood, tested and unbroken, and in doing so, it radiates isdom, tenacity, compassion, and resolve on every page. Sparta's Leonidas as right. A mother's strength is the warrior's ultimate inspiration."

–*Colonel Paul McHale (US Marine Corps, Ret.), former congressman and former as- tant secretary of defense*

"These mothers are heroes in their own right. They have given so much and we must never forget."

—*Gary Sinise, award-winning actor and philanthropist, founder of the Gary Sinise Foundation, and a champion of service members, veterans, and their families*

"The Mighty Moms and their wounded warriors featured in this remarkable book have sacrificed so much for our freedoms. *Unbreakable Bonds* is a touching testament to their strength and resolve, and is a must-read for anyone who values the power and perseverance of the human spirit."

—*Colonel Bob Clement, former congressman (D-TN), US Army (Ret.)*

"This is a book about courage, about service, and about patriotism. It is a call to arms, because we are in many ways failing a group of heroes that needs our support desperately. And, most importantly, it is an inspiring look at the strength that comes from the unbreakable bond of love and devotion. This is the kind of book that will have you talking, feeling, and thinking for a long time after you turn the last page."

—*Peter M. Weichlein, CEO of the US Association of Former Members of Congress*

"This book reminds us that we are all in this fight together. It will bring tears of sorrow, but mostly joy. I hope everyone gets to know these truly amazing moms and their real-life heroes."

—*Dennis Hertel, former congressman (D-MI), founder and vice president of Global Democracy Initiative, cochair of the FMC annual Wounded Warrior Charity Golf Tournament*

"These brave men and women are our heroes, and to their families, you are all heroes as well! Without the love and support of the families, the work of the soldier could not be done."

—*Betty D'Agostino Trimble, mother of Grammy Award–winning country singer Tim McGraw, who in 2013 teamed up with Operation Homefront and Chase Bank to provide mortgage-free homes to wounded warriors*

UNBREAKABLE
BONDS

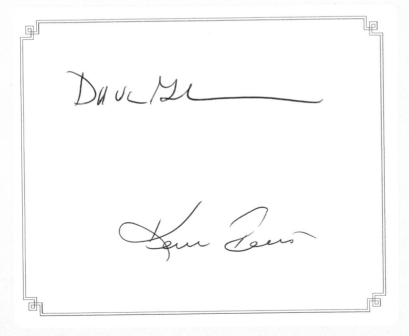

UNBREAKABLE BONDS

THE MIGHTY MOMS AND WOUNDED WARRIORS OF WALTER REED

Dava Guerin and Kevin Ferris
Forewords by President George H. W. Bush and Connie Morella

Skyhorse Publishing

Skyhorse Publishing books may be purchased in bulk at special discounts for sales promotion, corporate gifts, fund-raising, or educational purposes. Special editions can also be created to specifications. For details, contact the Special Sales Department, Skyhorse Publishing, 307 West 36th Street, 11th Floor, New York, NY 10018 or info@skyhorsepublishing.com.

Skyhorse® and Skyhorse Publishing® are registered trademarks of Skyhorse Publishing, Inc.®, a Delaware corporation.

Visit our website at www.skyhorsepublishing.com.

10 9 8 7 6 5 4 3 2 1

Library of Congress Cataloging-in-Publication Data is available on file.

Back cover photo credit © Josh Ghering

A portion of the proceeds of the sales of the book will be donated to each mom and her wounded warrior.

Print ISBN: 978-1-62914-698-0
Ebook ISBN: 978-1-63220-166-9

Printed in the United States of America

This book is dedicated to Mighty Moms everywhere, especially Ellene Fleishman, my mom. They paved the way for the ten remarkable women in this book, and their equally inspiring wounded warrior sons and daughter. I was inspired, too, by my father—the late Dr. Martin Lewis Fleishman, an Army Air Corps pilot during World War II, and my husband, Terry Bivens, a proud veteran of the US Coast Guard. Stacy Fidler, Mark Fidler, and Kelly Fidler were the genesis for writing this book, and Gary Sinise showed by example that one individual can truly make a difference. Finally, President George H. W. Bush and Barbara Bush are national treasures, and champions of what is most important in life—service, patriotism, family, faith, and friendship.

—Dava Guerin

For all the Blue Star, Silver Star, and Gold Star Moms, and for Frances Mary Strong Ferris.

—Kevin Ferris

ACKNOWLEDGMENTS

THIS BOOK WAS A JOY AND HONOR TO WRITE FOR SO MANY REASONS. IT has been an honor to get to know these ten truly courageous and inspirational Mighty Moms and their wounded warrior sons and daughter. They have shared their lives with us—warts and all. We have cried together, laughed together, and spent countless hours talking about their experiences as caregivers of some of the most catastrophically injured soldiers and Marines. Without them, this book would never have taken shape, nor serve as a record of their struggles and triumphs.

It all began with Chelle McIntyre-Brewer, who has a nonprofit organization that helps wounded warriors called Socks for Vets. She suggested a visit with Corporal Mark Fidler, three months after he was injured in Afghanistan. One visit with Mark on Valentine's Day 2011 at Walter Reed in Bethesda, Maryland, was all it took. He was the inspiration for this book, and he continues to inspire everyone he touches with his humor and defiance. It comes as no surprise that his mother, Stacy, shares that same strong will and keen intelligence. Through the love and devotion to her son, and her advocacy on behalf of all of the Mighty Moms, she served as the genesis for the book and its theme. We thank Stacy for the inspiration. Her daughter, Kelly, was an invaluable resource. She contributed her editing skills to the project, and helped us understand what it means to be a family member of a wounded warrior. Mark's father, Kermit, has supported us, as well as his sister, Amanda, who is a joy to know. We want to thank Mark's brother, Dan, a chief warrant officer in the Marine Corps, and his wife, Brittney, for their service and sacrifice, too.

From the start, Gloria Camma, our executive assistant, has used her administrative skills to keep the project on track. Ellene Fleishman spent countless hours editing the book and making some excellent editorial observations. Retired Army Colonel Dan Georgi helped us understand some of the military terminology, as did Navy Chief Warrant Officer Ron Carpenter, whose encouragement was most appreciated. Pete Weichlein provided many hours of support and guidance, and offered the tremendous brain power of the US Association of Former Members of Congress as a resource.

Jean Becker, President George H. W. Bush's chief of staff, generously offered expertise throughout the project, not to mention her humor and support. Our attorney, agent, and friend Lloyd Remick guided us and was a source of great insight. We were also inspired by the wonderful folks at Operation Homefront—Jim Knotts and Felecia Suluki—who introduced us to some of the Mighty Moms; Jennifer Brusstar of the Tug McGraw Foundation, who introduced us to Operation Homefront, coordinated our photo shoot, and generously offered her insights and experience; and Carol Harlow of the Elizabeth Dole Foundation for its work supporting caregivers.

Paulette Mason used her marketing and communications skills to improve every facet of the book. Gary Sinise and the Gary Sinise Foundation, along with the foundation's executive director, Judy Otter, have helped so many service members and their families, including our Mighty Moms and their warriors. Gary is a real American hero.

We would also like to thank the following people for providing their interest, expertise, and advice: bestselling authors Mark Bowden and Peter Collier; editors extraordinaire William Kristol of the *Weekly Standard* and William K. Marimow of the *Philadelphia Inquirer*; and friends and writers J. Christian Adams, Christine M. Flowers, and Jonathan V. Last of the *Weekly Standard*. The *Inquirer* published an essay about Mark and Stacy on Mother's Day 2013, and the positive response helped solidify the Mighty Moms' theme. We also want to acknowledge those who read early drafts or otherwise offered support, including Orlando R. Barone, Hunter Bivens, Nick Bivens, Roseann Costantino, Emily Ferris, Gerard Ferris, Richard Fleishman, Gabrielle Fleishman, Rachel Haas, Sharon Willis Holland, Jodie Chester Lowe, Irma Murphy, Mike Norris, Selma Robey, Amy and David Shepard, Mary Spivak, Kristen Waterfield, Estelle Weinstein, Sheldon Fleishman, and Sharon Witiw.

A very special thanks to Dr. Bonnie Burnquist, a retired Air Force Lieutenant Colonel who specializes in internal medicine and provided expertise, encouragement, and compassion. We are also deeply grateful to Jenny Pierson, our wonderful editor at Skyhorse Publishing.

We would like to thank Terence Ford, distinguished photographer and instructor for the Tug McGraw Foundation (TMF) fStop Warrior Project, and Marine Staff Sergeant Josh Ghering, who generously donated their time to photograph our book's back cover, and took portraits of our Mighty Moms and their wounded warriors. The program helps rehabilitate our nation's heroes through the art of photography with a year-long course that supports the recovery and transition of veterans with post-traumatic stress disorder and traumatic brain injury.

Finally, we vigorously salute all veterans who have fought for our country. Their service will be remembered in the hearts and minds of those who loved them, and all of us who reap the benefits of their sacrifice.

TABLE OF CONTENTS

FOREWORD

President George H. W. Bush

AT ABOUT AGE EIGHTY-FIVE, I DECIDED TO GIVE UP A NUMBER OF THINGS, including writing forewords for books. For the most part, I felt I had run out of interesting things to say.

It is my privilege to break that pledge for this remarkable book, *Unbreakable Bonds: The Mighty Moms and Wounded Warriors of Walter Reed*. In ways that are both heartbreaking and yet uplifting, *Unbreakable Bonds* celebrates two groups of heroes whom I pray for every night: wounded warriors and mothers.

Every commander in chief before and after me would agree that working with our military is the single biggest privilege of being president of the United States. There is no harder decision we face than to put our men and women in harm's way; and there's no worse news to receive than that someone has been killed or injured.

Unfortunately, too many Americans forget the sacrifices that our troops are making every single day until we see the coffins carried off a military plane at Dover Air Force Base, or see occasional publicity about wounded warriors projects and fund-raisers.

This is why this book is so timely and so important. It also is unique, telling our wounded warriors' stories through the eyes of their mothers— the remarkable strong women to whom they come home, and who instill in their sons and daughters the belief that life still holds for them great joy and potential. I have had the privilege of knowing many remarkable mothers—including my daughter and daughters-in-law—but two women of course stand out: my mother, Dorothy Walker Bush, who taught me so much about what is important in life; and my wife of sixty-eight years, Barbara Pierce Bush, who raised five remarkable children. Gratefully, neither of them had the challenges faced by the mothers in *Unbreakable Bonds*, yet I see their enduring strength and love in these mothers' stories.

I am grateful to the authors, Kevin Ferris and our friend Dava Guerin, for allowing all of us to share in these families' very personal journeys.

One last thought: tonight, when you go to sleep, remember that at this moment there is a young man and woman halfway around the world, sitting alone in the dark, waiting to go out on patrol. They may be tired, and even a little scared, but every day they put on that uniform and they lay their lives on the line for each of us, and for the United States of America. Say a prayer that they come home safe and sound.

George H. W. Bush
41st President of the United States of America
Houston, Texas, January 2014

FOREWORD

Connie Morella (R-MD)

I HAVE BEEN PRIVILEGED TO SERVE AS A MEMBER OF CONGRESS FROM MARY-land and as US ambassador to the Organization of Economic Coopera-tion and Development (OECD). My public service has been meaning-ful to me, but I consider my most important role that of being a mother.

That is why I am pleased to recognize this wonderful book: *Unbreak-able Bonds: The Mighty Moms and Wounded Warriors of Walter Reed*. These ten remarkable women, and their wounded warrior sons and daughter, inspire Americans to cherish their own children. Let us celebrate the strength of these selfless women who gave up everything to care for their young heroes who tragically became victims of the wars in Iraq and Afghanistan. Caring for injured children, especially young adults who are independent and are pursuing their own lives, can be daunting. But the Mighty Moms show us that when it comes to loving their children, there are no limits. This is their call to duty.

I know firsthand how difficult their struggles have been. My sister passed away from a long battle with cancer, leaving behind six young children. With three children of our own, there was not a moment of doubt regarding who would raise them. My husband and I adopted all of my sister's children, and today our loving family is a unit with unbreakable bonds as well.

As president of the US Association of Former Members of Congress—dedicated to service, dialogue, and bipartisanship—I've had the opportunity to meet brave wounded warriors through events we host that support them.

When I see how these Mighty Moms embrace their young heroes, and do whatever it takes to help them get through their ordeal, I am in awe! They inspire me every day, and I feel a special bond with them because of their unwavering tenacity and strength.

Unbreakable Bonds is a book that I hope will be read by every American. As a nation, we will always honor our brave wounded warriors, and at the same time, celebrate the strength and love of their Mighty Moms.

Connie Morella (R-MD)

Bethesda, Maryland, January 2014

INTRODUCTION

*U*NBREAKABLE BONDS: THE MIGHTY MOMS AND WOUNDED WARRIORS *of Walter Reed* is based upon the remarkable stories of ten young wounded warriors who have been treated at the Walter Reed National Military Medical Center, and their devoted mothers who have become their caregivers. (The medical center was established on November 10, 2011, when the Department of Defense consolidated the Bethesda Naval Hospital and National Naval Medical Center and Walter Reed Army Medical Center.) These young service members suffered extreme injuries from improvised explosive devices (IEDs), small-arms fire, and other perils of the wars in Iraq and Afghanistan. Once independent, these young men and women have had to rely primarily on their mothers to dress their wounds, administer medications and shots, help them in and out of their wheelchairs, take them to endless medical appointments and surgeries, and become their constant companions. At a time when they should have been starting lives of their own, they spent weeks and months in hospital beds, always within sight of loved ones who vigilantly watched over them.

The lives of their moms—Silver Star Mothers, as they are known—have changed dramatically as well. Now they are caregivers to their adult children, experiencing the same difficulties as any caregiver would, giving up the comfort of their homes, losing their jobs, suffering from physical and mental fatigue, and not knowing what the future holds. But to the Mighty Moms of wounded warriors, just like all mothers and their children, their bonds are unbreakable and timeless. Together, they face the future with determination and hope, despite the constant struggles to adjust to life without arms and legs, and with scars both physical and psychological. Their strength is an inspiration to anyone who has the good fortune to become part of their lives.

It is estimated that more than 50,000 US service members have suffered visible injuries and more than 250,000 have suffered invisible wounds, including traumatic brain injuries and post-traumatic stress disorder, as a result of the wars in Iraq and Afghanistan. But the price paid by their caregivers has been substantial, too. A RAND study entitled "Hidden Heroes: America's Military Caregivers," commissioned by the Elizabeth Dole Foundation and released in April 2014, reports that there are 5.5 million wives, husbands, siblings, parents, children, and friends caring for wounded veterans—with 1.1 million of those caregivers who are looking after war fighters injured after the terrorist attacks on September 11, 2001. Because of the seriousness of the wounds involved, those caring for their warriors often experience more stress, as well as physical and mental health problems, than their civilian counterparts.

As the wars wind down, the news coverage will no doubt abate. And as the war fighters return home, public awareness of their sacrifices may also fade. Many of our brave wounded warriors, however, are left with permanent injuries and will be dependent on the military medical system and their loved ones for the rest of their lives. That is why their very personal stories need to be told and why their sacrifices must never be forgotten by the American public.

The stories in the book also showcase the selfless love and support of the mothers who, like their wounded warriors, have been changed forever, and who have, without hesitation, sacrificed greatly for their precious sons and daughters. They bear these burdens heroically, knowing that their children's care is their number one priority. These sacrifices cannot be underestimated.

Many of the Mighty Moms have lost their jobs and their homes and have faced severe financial hardships. Their personal relationships have suffered, too. Marriages have been strained or dissolved, and friends often have a difficult time relating to what they go through. Even when their marriages are strong, long separations and the challenges of taking care of their wounded warriors often negatively affect even the best of personal situations. Worse, some caregivers bear the additional burden of watching their wounded warriors deal with issues beyond their wounds: wives, husbands, stepparents, or girlfriends who walk away when they can't handle the new reality; intimacy issues; substance abuse; spouses betraying their warriors; financial problems; divorce and custody battles; and even questioning whether life is still worth living.

The Mighty Moms find great strength and compassion through their exclusive network of caregivers, who support not only their sons and daughters, but each other as well. They make sure no mom who arrives at Walter Reed is alone. They know firsthand the value of institutional knowledge and experience, and pass theirs along to new caregivers. They work together as a team to ensure that no mom is left behind. Their contribution is immeasurable. According to the Family Caregiver Alliance and the National Center on Caregiving, "Caregiving is the backbone of the American long-term care system: the value of the services provided by informal caregivers (family or friends of seriously ill loved ones) is estimated at $306 billion annually."

We hope readers will not only learn about the real impact of war on wounded warriors, but also be inspired by the courage and determination of mothers as they confront their children's horrific injuries. Readers will come to appreciate the sacrifices the warriors and their loved ones make in support of our country and, as a result, support them in their transition from battlefield to home front, and be inspired to dedicate their own lives to service and helping others.

In addition, these stories will illustrate some of the signature wounds of the Iraq and Afghanistan wars and the ways military medicine has kept these heroes alive. Readers will experience the struggles and triumphs of the wounded warriors' rehabilitation, and get to know "Building 62," where they live at Walter Reed. They will also learn how the Mighty Moms use their considerable skills to advocate for their children and support one another, and how humor plays a role in their warriors' recovery. Finally, there is a list of nonprofit organizations that, according to the Mighty Moms, provide the best services for wounded warriors and their families.

These stories are not intended to be the last word on the wars in Iraq and Afghanistan, nor a comprehensive history of the times in which they were waged. They are memoirs told from the point of view of families, in particular the moms, who are heroically coping with the consequences of those wars.

Ultimately, we hope these stories will serve as a reminder that people with disabilities are just like everyone else. They should not be defined by their injuries, but by how they live their lives.

Award-winning actor and philanthropist Gary Sinise, founder of the Gary Sinise Foundation and a champion of service members, veterans, caregivers, and their families, perhaps said it best:

"I have visited our military hospitals many, many times since our country began deploying troops in reaction to the September 11, 2001, attacks. Thousands have been wounded in Iraq and Afghanistan. On every one of my visits I have met mothers whose sons or daughters lay in hospital beds trying to recover, and I have always been humbled by the strength and resiliency of these incredible women. In some cases they will be the only caregiver who will never leave the bedside. All of them are determined to do whatever it takes to ensure the best for their children as they go through months, and in many cases years, of rehabilitation. As I continue the mission to give back to these families, all I have to do is think about our wounded warriors and the mothers who care for them and I am inspired and reenergized to do whatever I can to support them. These mothers are heroes in their own right. They have given so much, and we must never forget."

ONE

MARK FIDLER AND STACY FIDLER

OTHER'S DAY IS TRADITIONALLY A TIME WHEN CHILDREN OF ALL AGES contemplate the gifts they will give their moms to celebrate the annual ritual. From flowers and jewelry, to perfume and spa days, Mother's Day gifts are cherished symbols of their children's love. But for one Pennsylvania mom—Stacy Fidler—a pair of legs, a motorized track wheelchair, or wounds that heal are even better. For the proud moms of our nation's wounded warriors, Mother's Day is a time to celebrate their children's sacrifices, and their solidarity as a group of unexpected heroines themselves.

October 3, 2011, was without question the worst day of Stacy Fidler's life. Far away from his Pennsylvania hometown, her son, US Marine Corps Lance Corporal Mark Fidler, twenty-two, took one fateful step that triggered an IED and changed his life forever.

As the proud mother of two sons who serve in the Marine Corps, Stacy has lived with the danger of military service for years, but she also knows that service is a calling, and the commitment that her sons hold is sacred. She couldn't think of another line of work nobler or more suited to her boys. Her oldest son, Dan, is a warrant officer. Stacy always knew he would take care of himself and be "fine." For Mark, that was a different story.

"I never worried about Dan," she said. "But Mark was always rambunctious, and lived his life on the edge. We always feared that he would be the one who would step on an IED. He would be the one who would be blown up."

And you can see that devil-may-care quality in his engaging smile and piercing gaze. Full, brown, and sparkly, his eyes tell a story of a young man filled with exuberance, and a lust for living—someone not at all afraid of taking risks. Mark embraces life with irreverence too. Don't tell him he can't do something. He will always prove you wrong.

"When Mark was thirteen, he broke both of his legs in a car accident and spent ten weeks in a wheelchair and then on crutches," Stacy said.

Before he joined the Marine Corps, he used to joke that he wanted to lose both of his legs so he could get the running prosthetic legs and be able to run like a Paralympian. "And," Stacy said, "when I would be milking the cows at the farm where I work, he would tell me, playfully, that he would rather have his feet cut off than to have to step in dog poop like me! So oddly enough, it didn't surprise us that, just two weeks into his first deployment, that's exactly what happened."

Mark dreamed of being a United States Marine all of his life. "That's all I ever wanted to do," he said, "and since I was a little kid I would imagine myself helping to defend our country. Getting the bad guys and keeping America safe were all I ever wanted to do."

He was destined for the job. Shooting guns, hunting, and fishing were as commonplace to Mark as eating and sleeping. His father, Kermit, a US Marine himself, and a Vietnam veteran, loves the outdoors. He currently owns a Pennsylvania buck farm called "Fidler's Whitetails," where he raises those majestic animals and hosts groups of avid hunters who get to see them in their glorious natural habitat.

Mark was up to the task, too. Armed with excellent marksmanship skills, a family history of service to the United States, and a burning desire to fight the bad guys, he couldn't wait until his first deployment. After he enlisted, he went through basic training and was assigned to a security detail in Washington, DC, not that far away from his family home in Strausstown, near Reading, Pennsylvania. In this small town, without a single traffic light, everyone knew the Fidlers, and Mark always made an impression.

"Mark was the kind of kid you just never forget," Stacy said. "He always wanted to be in the middle of the action, and didn't like not being in the fight."

After his assignment at the Marine base at Eighth and I Streets in Washington, he completed his training for combat duty at Twentynine Palms, in California, and was scheduled to deploy to Afghanistan. On September 11,

2011, as Stacy dropped Mark off at the airport, she had a feeling of dread. She remembered those seemingly playful encounters, where mother and son joked about being a Paralympian runner. As she watched Mark sitting quietly on the airport bench, she wanted to take a picture of him, thinking that this might be the last time she saw her son with both legs. "I was very nervous, and remember thinking to myself that I should get out of the car and take a picture," she said. "But I just drove away."

Mark Fidler arrived in Afghanistan on September 23. Just eleven days later, on October 3, while on foot patrol in Sangin, with a belt of 40 mm grenades strapped to his waist, Mark stepped on an IED. For Stacy, his devoted mother; his father, Kermit; his brother, Dan, and his wife, Brittney; his two sisters, Kelly and Amanda; and Amanda's husband, Bill, their lives would be inexorably changed in ways they would have never imagined.

"When we first got the phone call that Mark was injured, we really didn't know how serious it was," said Stacy. When a service member is wounded, communications are shut down to make sure the family is notified first, and doesn't find out about their children's injuries on social media sites or by any other external means. "We tried to get as much information as possible from his buddies and the doctors because Mark was unconscious. To this day he has no memory of the blast at all."

Eventually, the family would learn the details of what they now refer to as his "alive day." Mark was on a 6:00 a.m. foot patrol on the way back to his base, with the Marines who would be relieving his squad that morning. About 200 yards from the base, Mark, who was the fourth Marine in line, stepped directly on the IED; the metal detector had missed the device.

Mark, with twelve live grenades strapped to his waist, literally was blown up. The violent blast blew off both of Mark's legs, the right at the knee and the left just above the knee. Three of the grenades detonated, adding to the severity of his injuries. Most of the soft tissue around his lower back and buttocks was blown off. One of Mark's buddies frantically ran over to him, trying desperately to control his bleeding. As he was applying a tourniquet, he wasn't sure if Mark would live or die. In fact, Mark's heart did stop beating. His condition was so grave that the medical helicopter barely took the time to land. Mark was hoisted aboard. He was flown to Bastion, where he received 120 units of blood, then to nearby Bagram Air Base. Not long after, he was sent to Landstuhl Regional Medical Center in Germany. The center, near the US air base at Ramstein, is America's largest overseas medical facility. Once his condition was stabilized, Mark was transferred to Walter Reed.

"I first got that dreaded call from Kermit, and then I called my son Dan who also found out some of the details of Mark's injury at that time," said Stacy. "I remembered thinking that if just his legs were blown off that wouldn't be so bad, because then Mark could finally get those running legs. We were so hopeful that was the case."

At twenty-two years old, this strapping, rambunctious young man became another casualty of the War on Terror, and his fifty-two-year-old mom a caregiver for life.

For Stacy, family means everything.

Stacy used to love to see her boys come home; it was better than the alternative. Yet every mother of a US service member knows that risk comes with the job. After all, they volunteered to fight for their country. On holidays, when Mark, Dan, and the rest of the Fidler family gathered in their rural home, Stacy spoiled them in traditional Pennsylvania Dutch style. There was a feast, of course, complete with a special dish of mashed potatoes made with sugar and stuffing, which she playfully named "Fidler's Filling," and more food than anyone, even hungry Marines, could hope to devour. But after Mark was injured, the warmth of family, and the smell of a roast in the oven, was, sadly, replaced by tubes, drains, and monitors, and an ICU that took their breath away.

"We waited for Mark to arrive, and Dan was the first person to see him," Stacy said. "When we finally were able come into the room, it was absolutely terrifying! There was my precious boy, lying there, tubes everywhere, and completely unconscious. The ICU is a very frightening place to be, especially when it is your son, and you have no idea of what is going on."

As the family waited, bit by bit they learned how severe Mark's injuries really were. Though relieved he was receiving the critical care he needed, they understood that Mark had undergone severe trauma, and they were not sure if he was going to live or die.

Stacy's inner "mama grizzly" kicked in, and from that day on she became tougher than the toughest drill instructor, and a fierce protector of her now wounded warrior son.

"After the initial shock, I did what any other mom would do, spending days in the ICU, sleeping wherever I could, and checking Mark's vital signs on the monitors incessantly," Stacy said. "I remember watching that monitor endlessly just to see him breathe, yet never fully understanding how grave his injuries really were."

As Mark's doctors performed surgeries each day to try to save what was left of his legs, Stacy knew things weren't going well. His trauma surgeon finally had to break the news to the family. Mark would have both of his legs disarticulated at the hip, and the tissue from his legs would be used to rebuild the lower part of his back that was blown off during the blast. With no stumps to attach prosthetic legs to, Mark was an unlikely candidate for artificial legs.

"Because of Mark's particular case," said Stacy, "at this point having prosthetic legs would be awkward and would take a lot out of him. It's not like he can just pop them on in the morning and walk down the street."

All this proud Marine mom could do was cry.

But over the next few months, Stacy drew strength from Mark, and also had the support of her family, the Marine Corps, a host of other organizations, and of course, the other Mighty Moms of Walter Reed.

"Mark would always say, 'It is what it is, Mom,' but Mark and all these guys are not like most people," Stacy said. "We always talk about the fact that it seems like the service members who have the hardest time after a catastrophic injury like Mark's are the ones who think nothing will ever happen to them. Mark always thought he would lose his legs, and while it doesn't mitigate the pain, it helps him and all of us because we know his life will be just as full and productive as it was before the blast."

Over the next year, Mark would face a host of unexpected complications, and Stacy, and at times her other family members, would call Walter Reed home, a far cry from the bucolic life they led before the blast.

"Mark spent six months in the hospital, and there were so many ups and downs," said Stacy. "Just when I thought things were getting better, Mark had a seizure and was sent back to the ICU. He spent one month there, and then was finally brought back to the fourth floor of the hospital, and we were so happy that on November 10 he was awarded a Purple Heart."

One of the horrible ironies of war is the medical breakthroughs in trauma care that have their roots in military medicine. From robotic prosthetics to wound care and rehabilitation advancements, long-term survival rates and quality of life have dramatically improved. For wounded active duty service members—and there are nearly two thousand who have lost limbs in Iraq and Afghanistan—being treated at Walter Reed has made all the difference.

"There is no question that Mark would have died if not for his buddy helping him at the scene, and Dr. Patrick Basile, who put his body back together like a jigsaw puzzle," Stacy said. "Dr. Basile literally used my son's legs to cover the soft tissue that was lost, and he was also part of the team, along with Dr. Potter, who just completed the first double-arm transplant on another patient. Thanks to him, Mark was also successfully treated for a condition called heterotopic ossification, where after a blast injury like Mark's, bone grows where it shouldn't, and that creates unbearable pain."

Stacy and her family were there at every stage of his treatment and recovery. When he first arrived, he was immediately assigned an active duty liaison who did everything for Mark, including carrying him to and from the ambulance, visiting him every day, helping with paperwork, and taking care of any need the family had. The military also provides a recovery care coordinator and a nurse case manager. A military liaison makes sure everyone is working together. In addition, the Armed Services Foundation pays for food and lodging, and a host of other support groups, including the Semper Fi Fund, Luke's Wings, Freedom Alliance, and the Yellow Ribbon Fund, helps with everything from buying a Sleep Number bed and track wheelchairs, to paying for flights for family members and providing families with a much-needed free trip or a dinner out of the hospital environment.

"I am blessed to have a very supportive family, and all of my children and their spouses were there for us from the very beginning of this ordeal," Stacy said. "Dan's wife and Amanda's husband were so giving of their time, and without them, and all my children, I don't know how I would have made it through."

Despite the assistance of so many people, the hospital is a far cry from the comforts of home. During Mark's in-patient stay, Stacy spent most of her time in his room, which was covered from floor to ceiling with photos, American flags, Marine memorabilia, and cards from many well-wishers. There was lots of food, too. In fact, Stacy complains that she gained at least fifteen pounds from her lack of exercise, and from eating all of the candy and cookies that filled his hospital room. After all, her mission was to help Mark recover, both physically and mentally. So, day after day, night after night, she claimed the corner of that room, taking turns with Mark's dad, as her temporary home, sleeping on a small, uncomfortable cot, squeezing in showers when she felt she could leave Mark alone for a couple of minutes. Even for this experienced farmhand, it was a tough way to live. Through it all, she continued to be thankful that Mark was still alive, and that she was not a Gold Star Mother.

He was also in a great deal of pain, though he rarely complained. For a Marine, this was part of the job. While he was beginning to improve, the skin flaps and wounds from his many surgeries still were not healing properly.

"Sometimes it feels like I am walking on hot coals, but I don't have any legs or ankles," said Mark. "I have learned that is called phantom pain, and I just have to deal with it." He also is constantly hot, sweating profusely at times, and rarely ever feeling cool. He explains it this way: "Since I don't have any legs, there is less of my body that can dissipate heat, so I feel hot most of the time. One of the best days I have had since the blast was when I went on a trip with my family and got to float in a lake. I felt so free, and for a moment, forgot about the fact that I have no legs."

Mark also said that he still doesn't remember the details of the blast. "I just remember going to bed the night before and then waking up three weeks later in the hospital," he said.

As the months passed, Mark had his ups and downs—excruciating pain, high fever, infection, and more surgeries. Stacy and all of the Fidler family were there for him, though Stacy was his primary caregiver. Fortunately, her boss was willing to give her the time she needed to care for Mark, and she did try to go home to Strausstown to work on the farm when she could.

"Most people don't know what this is like unless you are living it every day," she said. "Mark wanted me here all of the time, because he was on so much medication that his memory was affected. It is very important to be an advocate for your son, and little things like making sure his medication is in order, or that his specialized bed is made properly, are extremely important."

Stacy also was a quick study when it came to Mark's medical care. She became the gatekeeper of his hospital room, monitoring who could come in and out, depending on how Mark felt at the time. "Walter Reed is a wonderful place, and there is no better hospital in the world to care for the grave injuries Mark suffered. But sometimes, it was hard for him to have groups of doctors staring at him, or having celebrity visitors come in. They all mean well, but sometimes I had to graciously let them know that Mark simply wasn't up for their visits."

And everyone wants to help, a very good thing, according to Stacy. Wounded warriors do garner a good deal of attention and admiration for their sacrifice, as they should. Frequent visitors to Walter Reed include President Barack Obama and First Lady Michelle Obama, senators and congressmen, Prince Harry, and celebrities from Kid Rock and Bradley Cooper to regulars like Gary Sinise. And the guys really are happy to see them. On one visit to the hospital by an actor from the show *Psych*, Mark was overheard saying: "Thanks so much for coming to see me, man. But maybe you could stop and visit some of the other guys, too, because they have it much worse than me."

The fact is that very few guys did have it as bad as Mark, but once a Marine, always a Marine. Even after such catastrophic injuries, they still look after one another.

As the months progressed, Mark was well enough to be transferred to Building 62, which is the residence for wounded warriors and their families on the Walter Reed campus. A new facility, it not only contains wounded warrior housing, but also administrative offices, and a full-service restaurant called the Warrior Café on the first floor where wounded warriors and their caregivers, plus the plethora of military medical and civilian staff, chow down on the day's specials, salads, pizza, sandwiches, and other goodies.

Mark and Stacy live on the fourth floor of Building 62. On his hallway door is an American flag—most of the apartment doors have flags on them as well—and a Marine flag, too. Stacy has done everything she could to make the apartment feel like home, such as adding her collection of plants, posters on the walls, and books on the end tables, as well as a large leather sofa given to her by a relative. While it certainly isn't her comfortable home back in Strausstown, it is still a far better place to be than in the hospital itself. Only about 1,000 square feet, the apartment looks like it could be a spartan suite in a Holiday Inn, except for the odd sign above the toilet that reads: "Do not drink the water. Rainwater in use. Not suitable for consumption." Stacy explains that it is a "Navy thing."

Across the street, Mark and his fellow soldiers and Marines spend their days in endless physical therapy sessions, as well as classes, including how to drive a specialized car, live independently, manage pain while walking with prosthetic legs, function with robotic limbs, and a host of other, very necessary tasks to help them return to a normal life.

Most warriors living at Building 62 have lost something—an arm, a leg, two limbs, even four. Waiting in the lobby, there is a constant parade of motorized wheelchairs and Segways, and the clicking sounds of robotic limbs. But, for Mark and Stacy, they have gained so much, too—courage, patience, compassion, pride, and empathy.

"What is there to get depressed about?" said Stacy. "Mark will be fine. He actually does more hunting now than he has ever done before. People look at someone with a handicap and say, 'Gosh, look at what they can't do.' We look at them and say, 'Yes, they are handicapped, but look what they can do.'"

"I'm hoping to have my own car repair business when I get back home," Mark said.

"You know, I had a real blast in Afghanistan," he jokes, something only guys like him could get away with. Obviously one thing Mark has not lost is his wry sense of humor and biting wit. Some of the Mighty Moms have learned to take part in this "black amputee humor" too, making jokes about their sons' lack of arms and legs, or about why they don't need socks. Some have been even known to paint their sons' prosthetic legs when they weren't looking! And Stacy can match her son line for line. "You know, when Mark gets home, he'll be a worse pain than he was before. The only difference is that now he won't be raking up the leaves for me. I'll have to do it for him!"

On a more serious note, Mark really regrets being blown up only days into his first combat mission. "I wish I were able to do some real good in Afghanistan, and use all of my training to get the bad guys," said Mark. "Even though I lost my legs and have all these injuries, I would still do it all over again for my country."

While wounded warriors may be missing arms and legs and may need to do things differently, they can still do almost everything they did before. In fact, Mark shot an 800-pound elk from 600 yards away while on a hunting trip, and is collecting tools and building a heated garage, built by a local company, Pioneer Pole Buildings, where he can work on refurbishing classic cars.

Mark and Dan joined the military because their parents—Stacy and Kermit—raised them in a way that stressed love of country, commitment to service, and answering the call. Both parents inspired their sons in different ways.

Kermit served in the Marines at the height of the Vietnam War. Stacy loves her family and her country, and her patriotism and pride are evident to everyone she knows. Proof is in the military memorabilia on display in her home, but also the well-used copy of the US Constitution that she often carries with her, and her love of history. She knows the Bill of Rights almost verbatim.

Stacy is the embodiment of countless communities across the nation: solid, unassuming, and unpretentious, she accepts the tremendous challenge life has thrust upon her and simply gets the job done. Stacy has been the rock in her son's life, focusing 100 percent on his recovery. Unlike most young adults in the hospital, wounded warriors not only have to deal with devastating physical injuries, but with serious psychological ones as well. And moms can make all the difference.

Stacy and the other moms at Walter Reed have learned how to navigate the medical system, serving as their sons' and daughters' advocates and constant companions. While Stacy soldiers on, there is no doubt that at times she feels exhausted and frustrated. But, to her, Mark and all the other guys are real heroes. And when the inevitable moment of exasperation comes, she has a support group that knows 100 percent what she feels, fears, and needs. The Mighty Moms of Walter Reed band together, support each other, and protect one another—just like their children did when they were serving in Iraq or Afghanistan.

For the hundreds of moms like Stacy who are caring for their wounded warrior children, giving everything to help them recover is simply part of their job description. "You know I would do this for any one of my kids," Stacy said. "That is just what moms do."

But, most moms don't have to leave their homes and jobs and take care of their twenty-two-year-old sons. While some, like Stacy, work on a farm and live in rural areas, others are from large cities and work in offices, or are stay-at-home moms. In any case, they find themselves part of a new family—one that revolves around the care and rehabilitation of their wounded warriors.

Stacy, though petite and unassuming, isn't shy when it comes to Mark's medical care, and the care of the sons of her newfound friends at Walter Reed. She uses her intelligence and drive to advocate for many issues that she thinks will help the recovery of every wounded warrior. And she makes the time to do it, no matter how tired or exhausted she may be. Many of the soldiers and Marines spend years there, moving from the hospital, Building 62, and the other rehabilitation areas on base, to eventually going home or having a "smart house" built for them by organizations such as the Gary Sinise Foundation, Operation Homefront, and others.

"I never thought I would take care of my twenty-two-year-old son," said Stacy. "You literally give up your life when you move here, but I have a life and a home and other children, and grandchildren, and I plan on getting back there soon."

In the meantime, Mark relies on Stacy, and that is evident in their daily lives together. He asks her to check his medications, dress his wounds, get him things he can't reach, coordinate his outings, and scores of other things that most people take for granted. Most twenty-somethings, especially tough Marines, wouldn't be comfortable asking their mothers to help. Bonds like this are unanticipated, but they are forever.

"Mark and I were always close, and I guess you could say this experience has made us even closer," she said. "I would do this for any one of my other kids too, and all of the moms and wives here are doing the same thing for their loved ones as me." The truth is, without Stacy there by Mark's side, his prognosis might not have been so good. She was there 24-7 to monitor every aspect of his care, including making sure his wounds were healing, checking to see if he had a temperature, and even cooking his favorite meals. Teamwork really does pay off.

One of the surprising and rewarding aspects of this experience, according to Stacy, is the bond that is formed among the moms, and the lasting friendships that have come from a shared, unique experience. From the moment they come to the hospital, and throughout their stay, the Mighty Moms of Walter Reed have forged a more perfect union; they are now warriors in their own right.

But instead of spending their time in the hair salon, or dining at an outdoor café, they are together at benefit concerts, doctors' appointments, and fund-raisers. The future isn't cheap, and they must learn to navigate the system and rely on the generosity of others to assure their children can live independently somewhere down the road. These strong and determined women have traded in their conversations about fashion and recipes to ones about prosthetics and doctors.

"There are so many rewarding parts of this experience, but the most wonderful thing I ever heard was that I wasn't going to become a Gold Star Mom," said Stacy. "Once I realized that, I knew I had to do the best I could to help Mark, and also the other guys who have sacrificed so much for our country. Having the support and love of the other moms here has made a huge difference for me and Mark. We get together socially, and their kids are like my kids. And I've gotten so attached to so many of them that it is a real loss when they leave. These are truly remarkable people, and though we live in a kind of bubble here, it is a bubble I am so proud to be a part of.

"Very few people can understand what we are going through, and that's why we have formed such close relationships, and we know they will be long-lasting. We've become so strong as a group of women, and do things for each other like contacting our senators, or sharing information on what drug works, or which doctor we like, and we support each other no matter what! One time a Navy captain asked what he could do to help get these guys better, and I said, 'Just tell the world to accept these guys because there will be a lot of them out there missing body parts and dealing with disabilities.' They will see them in wheelchairs in their hometowns, and I want everyone to also know that they are wonderful, capable people. Wheelchairs are not just for older people."

Stacy admits that she may have a "big mouth," but she says that when one mom has an issue, "we all have an issue." Ultimately, they are bonded to one another, and they look out for each other as they would for their own families. Stacy even continues to attend the nonmedical attendant meetings, not because she wants to know what is going on, but to seek out other moms and wives, and offer them her advice and share her experience as a caregiver.

Mark is proud of his mom, too, as are her other children. He looks at her not as her dependent, but as a devoted, loving son. "My mom is really awesome," he said. "I guess I didn't really grow from this experience, I kind of shrank," he added with a laugh. "I am the person who I was before, and the same person I am now."

He's not a young man of many words—he doesn't have to say a thing! His eyes tell a story of strength, determination, caring, heart, perseverance, and most of all, what it means to be a son.

The following is a letter written to Lance Corporal Mark Fidler by President George H. W. Bush while Mark was recuperating at Walter Reed:

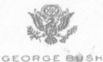

GEORGE BUSH

February 17, 2012

Dear Mark,

My friend Dava Guerin wrote me about her recent visit with you there at Walter Reed. She described the injuries you suffered and the difficulties you and all your family are facing as you deal with your recovery.

I don't pretend to know the trauma you have endured, Mark, and I wish there was something I could do to help. But maybe it does help a tiny bit to know that a lot of folks are in your corner praying for you and admiring you — and that includes Barbara and me. We have the highest regard for our men and women in uniform and their families, and we always remember them in our prayers and with gratitude in our hearts.

Hang in there, soldier. This Navy man and former Commander-in-Chief salutes you and sends you his respects and his warmest best wishes.

Sincerely,

G Bu

Lance Corporal Mark Fidler
United States Marine Corps

TWO

JOSH BRUBAKER AND MARY BRUBAKER

AYLON JENNINGS'S LEGENDARY COUNTRY SONG "MAMMAS DON'T Let Your Babies Grow Up to Be Cowboys" had an ironic twist for Mary Brubaker. Her son Josh, whose love of horses led him to compete in Cowboy Mounted Shooting Association events in Bakersfield, California, as well as all over the Midwest, always loved the cowboy lifestyle. But after college, this handsome, determined young man decided to trade in his six-shooter for an M-16. He joined the Marine Corps so he could rid the world of bad guys and use his criminal-justice degree in a way that would make a difference. After the tragic events of June 1, 2012, Mary sometimes wishes he would have grown up to be a cowboy after all.

Mary Brubaker, fifty-six, is a tall, striking woman with brown wavy hair and almost perfect diction. When she speaks, she commands attention. She has that special something—an indefinable quality that makes people want to listen. She lives in Bakersfield, and is the mother of four sons—all born two years apart—and one of whom is mentally challenged. Her husband, Bill, a harvest manager for Bolthouse Farms, spends many months of the year away from home. "Yes, carrots are big business," Mary explains. Josh is their second son, and since he was born, she knew they had a special connection. And one of their main shared passions is horses.

"We had a mini-ranch," Mary said. "At one point we had as many as twenty horses on a two-and-a-half-acre property. We sold and bred them, and also would train horses for people who knew we had that ability. When the economy soured, we decided to sell most of our horses, but did end up keeping four, including Josh's favorite—Peppy."

When Josh got involved in 4-H at age fourteen and went on one of their many field trips, he discovered the Cowboy Mounted Shooting Association, which boasts that it is the fastest-growing equestrian sport in the country. It was perfect for Josh. Not only must competitors be excellent riders, but they also have to be good with a gun. Josh was a natural at both. He would practice every day for at least four hours, using a .45 Long Colt, a single-action revolver with five rounds of specially loaded black powder ammunition to hit the targets—all on horseback.

Each horseman rides patterns that can change with every competition, and there are categories based upon age and skill level. Each round requires firing at ten balloons, and a pattern might consist of five red balloons and five white balloons, but they may be grouped together in different areas of the competition field. The goal is to shoot the five white balloons first, holster the first gun, and shoot the five red balloons with the second gun.

"I rode horses most of my life," Josh said. "Pistol shooting is very different from rifle shooting, which is what I used in the Marine Corps. In a combat situation you use a longer-range rifle, and, of course, you are using real bullets. When I am competing with my horse, we have a real partnership, and that makes a difference in the outcome. Precision shooting is a whole different beast. I can say, though, that when I enlisted in the Marines, I knew I had a lot to learn, and just kept my mouth shut and let them teach me because I needed to understand more. But the advantage of being a mounted shooter was that I was clearly not afraid of a gun."

That came in handy as Josh began his new life as a US Marine.

Mary told Josh he could not enter the Marine Corps unless he went to college and got a degree. "Josh wanted to be a Marine since he was a kid," Mary said. "It was all he wanted to do, and I told him that I would allow him to enlist and give him my blessing if he finished college."

He agreed, and enrolled in Taft College, earning an associate's degree in criminal justice in 2010. His dream was now within reach, and he visited the recruiter in Bakersfield soon after graduation. They were more than thrilled to have this driven, intelligent young man join the Corps.

Mary was very proud of Josh, like so many mothers whose children have served in the armed forces. Of course, she worried too, but she somehow believed that Josh's shooting skills and perfectionist personality would enable him to fight and still stay safe. "In January 2010, my son left for boot camp, and what a day with a lot of tears, especially when he was driving away from his family," Mary said. "I thought it couldn't get any worse than that moment; boy, was I wrong."

Josh trained at Camp Pendleton, which was only a few hours away from their home. After he graduated, he was assigned to the 2/5 Echo regiment, an amphibious assault group. "This was good news to me since there was no water in Afghanistan, so I thought things would be okay," said Mary. But after his first deployment, which was to Japan following the tsunami, he learned he would be heading to Afghanistan. His unit left on February 20, 2012, after desert warfare training at Twentynine Palms. "The boys were machine gunners so I knew they would be in the thick of things. I was proud of myself that I did not completely break down until I was back in the car and the boys could not see," Mary added.

The dreaded call came on June 1, 2012. Lance Corporal Josh Brubaker was on patrol in Helmand Province in Afghanistan when he stepped on an IED. The Marine on the other end of the line said Josh was in critical, but not life-threatening, condition. He was in surgery within only twelve minutes, and the pilot who flew him to safety holds the record for the fastest evacuation in Helmand Province, Mary was told.

Josh's injuries were extremely severe. His left leg was blown off below his knee. His right knee was shattered; he had major trauma to his pelvis, and soft tissue damage to his left hand.

For Mary, her husband, Bill, and the rest of the family, life would never be the same. "It was the worst day of my life, without a doubt," said Mary. "Josh was at the tail end of the mission, and he would have been coming home for good in only two more months. I was in shock, then disbelief, then more shock, and it took a while for it to really sink in."

Thousands of US service members have either stepped on IEDs or driven over them in Iraq and Afghanistan. When not fatal, IEDs cause severe injuries, leaving these brave men and women with a lifetime of physical and psychological challenges.

Getting treated at the scene, and then being quickly moved to a hospital, can mean the difference between life and death.

Josh was one of the lucky ones. After two surgeries in Afghanistan base hospitals, he was placed into a medically induced coma and immediately med-evacuated to the hospital in Landstuhl, Germany. "Fortunately, the Marines notified us every time Josh was okay to move to the next place. They talked to us about the details of him getting on the plane, his condition each step of the way, and answered many of our questions," said Mary. "It was great that the Marine Corps paid for our plane tickets to come to Bethesda."

Mary and Bill arrived in LA for the red-eye flight to the East Coast. The Marines met them at the airport, drove them to Walter Reed by 7:30 a.m., and took them to a meeting with other parents of the wounded. "I was not ready for that. I was on overload by this time and tired and nervous, and really scared," Mary recalled.

But Mary and Bill wouldn't lay their eyes on Josh until he came out of surgery at around 2:00 p.m. "We knew he lost his left leg below the knee, and that the blast ripped around the right side of his body. Unfortunately for Josh, he stepped on a dirty bomb, and as a result, developed a fungal infection, as well as a host of other ones," Mary said.

The three weeks Josh spent in intensive care were simply grueling for Mary. Every day she would look at her son, and sometimes she would just fall apart. "You have in your head that the doctors would just stitch them up and things would be fine," said Mary. "Just like a car accident, they would close up the wound and send them home. But I knew this wasn't going to be the case. It's hard to look at your kid when he is blown up. Not that having a disease is any easier, but this is unique. Sometimes I would remember when he was a little baby and I would tickle his toes. Now, I just miss those legs. But this is for real, and they are not coming back."

Day after day, week after week, Mary dutifully sat by Josh's side. She kept telling herself that things could have been much worse. Many moms of the wounded at Walter Reed will say they are thankful they never heard the "knock on the door": that they were not Gold Star Mothers.

"I used to have a terrible fear of leaving my house and that I would not be home when they knocked on my door," said Mary. "It was especially hard when Josh would call and say, 'I am going silent, Mom.' Now I wonder if this bad dream will ever end."

While in the ICU, Josh finally started to regain consciousness as he was removed from his medically induced coma. From the first time that Mary saw Josh after he returned from Afghanistan, she was ecstatic. "It was so good to see him that I think I didn't even notice the tubes and the wires or anything else at that moment. All I saw was that my son was alive, and he was the most beautiful sight I had ever seen!" That feeling would continue while he was in the ICU and through his move to the fourth floor of the hospital.

Once Josh woke up from the coma on June 6, he could not talk, but did respond to Mary by squeezing her hand. He was in a lot of pain, was heavily medicated, and had a massive cast on his left arm, a neck brace, and bandages on his waist and both legs. But, regardless, Mary was just happy that Josh was still alive, and most of all, thrilled to learn that he in fact did not suffer any traumatic brain injury. She also remembers the "Afghan Funk." Here's how she explains it: "I did notice after the initial shock that Josh was dirty and he had a very funky smell to him. They call it the 'Afghan Funk,' and let me tell you, it is really stinky!"

The second week that Josh was in the hospital, he received a visit he will never forget, according to Mary. "General Joseph F. Dunford came to see Josh on Wednesday and presented him with the Purple Heart. What a special day that was. I was so proud of my son; he had been through so much." Dunford was then assistant commandant of the Marine Corps.

There were lighter moments then too. "We laugh about this now, but as all of us know, these guys are on massive amounts of drugs like Dilaudid, Ketamine, and Propofol and can hardly function. I told Josh about some of the things he did and said in the hospital, and he remembers some of those very funny moments. Like when he was massively drugged up and said: 'Mom, I'm going on a trip and I'll be back.' His eyes would roll to the back of his head and he would be gone for a while. Then, he would wake up a bit later and tell me, 'Hi, Mom. I'm back.' We do crack up about that," Mary said, laughing.

"Then there was the time that the nurses came into Josh's room and they asked him about three questions, and also asked him to remember three words. They were clearly trying to gauge his level of awareness. The word could be a house, a dog, or a flower pot. Then they would talk to him for a bit, and ask him to remember those words they had mentioned, and asked him to repeat them. I thought, how could he answer all those questions with all of those drugs in him? Josh has never been on drugs his entire life, so this was completely a new experience for him. Later that same day, they blew my mind.

"They asked Josh to count back from one hundred, subtracting seven each time. I was furious. I firmly asked them to step outside with me and told them, 'Do you know the drugs that this kid is on right now? I can't do that and I am drug-free! And on top of that, you know he couldn't have done that even if he were on no drugs.' It is sometimes nuts."

There were even more serious incidents as Josh drifted in and out of his drug-induced fog.

At one point, as a nurse ran a thermometer across his forehead while he was asleep, Josh suddenly awoke, thinking someone was holding a gun to his head. He grabbed her arm and almost broke it. In his mind, according to Mary, he was being threatened and responded accordingly.

But the road to healing was far from over for Josh.

The day after General Dunford's visit, Josh's white blood cell count began climbing to a very dangerous level. The doctors told Mary that the level was as high as that of a person with end-stage cancer. Friday morning Josh went into surgery, and his doctor told Josh, Mary, and Bill that he had to make a choice. Lose his right leg or die. While the family was waiting for an operating room, Josh took a turn for the worse. His infection was spreading, and a trauma team was standing by. "I went to the chapel to pray for peace," Mary said, fearful of her son's most recent setback. "Not all moms get to hold their sons and tell them how much they love them. I was grateful for this time I had with him, so if it were to be that God was going to call him home, I was okay and I would survive, too."

The doctors were able to amputate the leg below the pelvis, ensuring that he would be able to be fitted for prosthetic legs. Dr. Michael Newman told the family that they had "one tough son."

Dr. Newman also said that they were not able to take care of the vascular issue Josh had, but they could do that the following morning. While he was on a twenty-four-hour watch, waiting for the surgery the next day, the unthinkable happened. Josh's artery ruptured, and Mary and Bill raced back to the hospital to a grueling sight. "I was not prepared for what I saw in his room," Mary said. "Everyone was covered in his blood; it was a mess. They wanted me to just talk to Josh and keep him calm, so they covered him up with clean towels and had me go stand by his head where he could see me." The trauma doctors were taking turns putting pressure on the ruptured artery, according to Mary. When the surgeons arrived at the hospital at around 4:00 a.m., Josh was taken to surgery. "The doctors said they had never seen a patient with such a low white blood cell count, but they performed the surgery and it went very well." Three days later, Mary got the news. His artery was repaired successfully, and his amputated right leg was on the mend. "Another miracle from God, I believe," Mary said. After reflecting on those trying times in the hospital, Mary had much to be thankful for.

"We are fortunate in that our sons and daughters are some of the most physically fit young people in the country, and so their bodies can handle more than the average population," said Mary. "Still, you don't realize the gravity of the situation until you almost lose them like I did with Josh. When he was in surgery to remove his leg, he flatlined on the operating table, and the next morning at 4:00 a.m. an artery burst in his right leg and we almost lost him. He remembers looking at the surgeon and felt like he was 'hovering over him,' which we kind of joke about now. You have to have a sense of humor sometimes, or this experience would be totally intolerable."

As the days and weeks passed, Mary was comforted by her close family and friends back home and the love and support of her fellow wounded warrior moms. Three weeks to the day that Josh arrived at Walter Reed, he finally left the ICU and was transferred to the fourth floor of the hospital. After three months there, Josh was released to the outpatient living quarters known as Building 62.

Building 62 feels like a hotel you might see when you are driving on the interstate. It's neat, tidy, and livable. There are lots of floors with long hallways and rooms flanked on either side—apartments, actually. There are no concierges or bellmen, just friendly folks in uniform who greet visitors and interact with the wounded warriors and their families.

In the lobby is the "freebie" table, where wounded warriors can take their pick from the gift of the day—CDs, razors, blankets, snacks, and whatever else is available as donations from nonprofit organizations or individuals. As the moms of Building 62 say, if your kid is blown up, he surely deserves whatever he can get to help him recover. Wounded warriors and their families are generally proud, independent people who hesitate to accept "freebies." When your mission is to serve others, it's difficult to be the recipient of the generosity of others, even with the new realities of injury.

While Building 62 is comfortable, and the two-bedroom apartment Mary shares with Josh is pleasant enough, it still can't compare with home. "Living here does get you down sometimes, it truly does," Mary said. "It isn't really home, and because we live 3,000 miles away, we can't go home to visit much, and, of course, friends and family visits are few and far between.

Sometimes Josh will ask me, 'Am I ever going to get well? Will I ever heal? Why do I have to be the odd duck and the one who can't heal?' I always tell him that even though you are watching guys up walking on their legs three months after they got here, someday you will have legs, too."

Josh's progress has been hampered not only by his injuries, but also by nagging fungal and bacterial infections. Many of his wounds, like those of most of the severely wounded warriors, require frequent skin grafts and complex procedures to keep the wounds from becoming infected and the new, delicate skin from breaking down. It is a slow process, and a seemingly endless waiting game. As Josh continues to receive specialized wound care and surgical procedures that will enable him to be fitted for prosthetic legs, Mary hopes and prays that his wounds will heal and he will be free of those nagging infections. "I know over time Josh will be up and walking, and while he will have issues for the rest of his life, he has an amazing spirit and tremendous determination. He is often my inspiration. We both knew that through all of this, God has a plan and it is going to be okay. There really is a light at the end of the tunnel."

Between his spirit and the excellent care Josh is receiving at Walter Reed, the Brubakers are beginning to understand the long-term challenges they face. "Before the blast, I really never thought about what it meant to be 'handicapped,' and it really never entered my mind," said Mary. "You never looked at that realm, and before you know it, you are forced to learn what a handicapped person really does need. You don't realize that certain things are just not accessible—like doorways that are too narrow for someone in a wheelchair to maneuver, or cabinets too high for them to reach things. Before, I took some things for granted, but now I realize how people with disabilities are no different from anyone else."

Others may see Josh differently now, but not his mom.

"Josh is the same terrific guy as he was before the injury. I tell him that he's got better legs than he had before, and his feet don't smell, either," she said jokingly.

"I tell people who look at us and feel sorry or sad, 'If you are going to cry, don't come in this door.' You need to have a sense of humor to keep yourself and your loved one on track. So I often remind Josh that before, he had those bird legs, and they were kind of scrawny, but soon he will have new ones that will look better in shorts."

One of the issues that most wounded warriors need to address is the sensitive subject of intimacy. Many of the blast victims are young men who have lost all or part of their genitals in the prime of their lives. Military medicine is addressing these issues with the wounded warriors and their caregivers, and some medical organizations that support them privately are also offering counseling.

"I know Josh and all of the guys think about their futures, and that includes getting married and having children, like any other normal young man. But they do have challenges they have to face in life, like intimacy. It is a big deal, and sometimes they look in the mirror and wonder if anyone would ever love them," Mary said.

Fortunately, these Mighty Moms and their sons can talk about anything. Their bonds are timeless, and their love and appreciation for each other's sacrifices is unbreakable.

Another of the major challenges for severely wounded warriors is relying so heavily on a caregiver, often a mom, at a time when others their age are independent.

"I guess you could say that Josh and I have very strong bonds, and that is sometimes good and sometimes bad. When he woke up from the coma, he said, 'Mom, are you going to stay with me?' He was never ashamed that his mom was taking care of him, but you have to acknowledge that they are young men, and who wants their mom to be taking care of them? These are extremely capable men who are willing to die for their country," Mary said.

"Of course it is always a struggle for independence, and Josh says he knows he will get it back someday, and that he isn't going to be dependent on his mom forever. As a caregiver and a mom, I must say I have grown a lot, and Josh and I, while we were always close, are now even more so. The truth is no one knows these guys better than us, and we know what they were like before, so we can anticipate problems before they happen or recognize them once they occur," she added.

"We get along so well," Josh said with a laugh. "But, it is hard to be dependent on someone else. The thing is I recognize I can't control it, so instead of fighting it, I accept it because I can't change things." He adds with a chuckle, "I can't wait to get away from my mom for at least two years."

"Seriously though," said Josh, "we have always had a strong bond, and while this thing kind of puts you in a weird spot, you have to just accept it. I mean, what would you think if you had to tell people that you and your mom are roommates? Sounds kind of weird. But, seriously, I don't know how my mom deals with this, but I knew she would always be able to handle whatever came her way." He said that when they were children, Mary had to handle Josh's brother almost losing a foot, and his other brother an arm, but he was the first one in the family to actually lose a limb.

"I'm sure the hardest thing for her was in the beginning, but I don't remember much from that time," Josh said. "But you definitely grow and learn from things like this, especially not letting little things get you down. Your family is what matters most, and I learned the importance of family from being with my mom. She is something else."

And there are other bonds that change lives, too. Bonds between strangers, thrown together by chance—all of whom share one common thread. Their sons and daughters are blown up, and they need to be there with them.

"There is not a mom in this place who wouldn't do the same thing for her son or daughter," Mary said. "Life is way too short, and we all find strength, not just from our kids, but also from the wonderful moms who are here with them. People will always tell me how strong I am, and I point out to them that I am not that strong; you would have done the same thing. We get that inner strength from each other because they all understand."

Mary said that she gets support from the many other moms who have been at Walter Reed for some time, as well as the new ones whom she and the others try to comfort. "We are our own best support and each other's sanity. We go for walks, or we will go on shopping trips, and we love getting away from here. Men hold in their feelings and we let them out, so having these strong women as friends has been a great blessing," Mary said. "It's been great to get to know women from all across the country, and their sons, too. Our bonds are so strong, and I hope they will last a lifetime. I also feel blessed to have the support of my husband, which not all of the moms here have. I think, now that I have been gone, he realizes just how much work around the house I really do. Now he is the one who has to do the laundry, take out the trash, cook the meals, and feed all of the animals."

"Most of the guys here who are with their moms are pretty motivated," Josh said. "There are a few guys who are really negative, and I tell them come back and talk to me when you are done pitying yourself. I want to help them, but they have to want to help themselves, first. And this experience has also made me realize how lucky I am to have the mom I have. Most guys have great moms, but one or two don't. Like one guy I know whose mom took money out of his bank account and gambled it all away. Fortunately, he is the exception."

For Josh and Mary the future is bright. "I have always loved law enforcement and that was my major in college," Josh said. "I want to work for the Drug Enforcement Agency, and already am applying for an internship, though people tell me I am overqualified. Can you believe that? But, I have talked to many federal agents, and they have been very encouraging. I also hope I will become an officer, and maybe have kids. I love Texas, and someday would love to live and work there."

Mary has some goals, too. "Our house is fairly accessible, and we will always want to make more changes to accommodate Josh. And, I was training my bloodhound, Fleas, to become a search-and-rescue dog before Josh was injured, so I'm hoping to be able to return to that when we go home. And, of course, I have quilts that have not been completed, and so many other things I want to do," Mary added. "I also hope to become a certified companion dog trainer. I want to give back to our warriors and be able to find and train whatever type of dog they may want, be it a small or large dog," said Mary.

Josh someday wants to get back on his horse. This time, he will compete in a different way, and his personal best will make him a winner.

While mamas may not want their sons to grow up to be cowboys, Mary is proud that her son grew up to be a Marine.

THREE

CHRISTIAN BROWN AND LYN BRADEN-REED

T HE 6:00 A.M. PHONE CALL THAT CHANGED LYN BRADEN-REED'S LIFE was brief and offered few details.

Her son, Christian Brown, a strapping US Marine on his second deployment to Afghanistan, had been wounded. Lyn would receive another call in twenty-four hours with more information and an update on his status. Those hours were excruciatingly long and frightening.

Finally, Christian's injuries were explained to her. While on foot patrol in Helmand Province with his squad on December 13, 2011, Christian had stepped on a pressure-plate improvised explosive device. The blast, Lyn said, "Blew him up in the air, and blew one half his body off with it."

As Christian recalls it, the day had been "eerie" from the start. What the Marines were used to as normal when pushing through the town was off: locals weren't in their usual spots, the reactions of the people to the troops' presence didn't feel right. The Marines moved into a building to reassess. When they were ready to leave, two Marines went through the doorway first, and Christian followed. He was about two feet from them when he hit the IED.

"We had all walked by it," Christian said. "Luck of the draw."

Bad luck for Christian.

Initially, Christian didn't realize what had happened. There had been an explosion. He was on his back. He was sure he needed to get up and help his Marines. He couldn't.

"I couldn't understand why I couldn't get my feet under me," Christian said.

When his buddies came to him, shouting, "I got you, I got you," he realized he'd been the one hit. They were scrambling to dress his wounds, tie tourniquets. He got a hint of how bad it was when he asked if his legs were still there. They wouldn't answer.

Then he was being pushed onto a medevac helicopter. Just six days earlier, Christian had been the one rushing a wounded Marine to a chopper.

Again, it had been a routine patrol. The Marines had gone into a building. They were preparing to evacuate the roof when Lance Corporal Jacob Levy, who as the senior Marine had stayed until the others were down, was shot in the head. "He buckled and fell into our arms," Christian said.

Seeing it was a critical wound, they called in for a chopper, trying to keep the enemy pinned down so it could land safely. But when the helicopter was about 10 feet from the ground, it unexpectedly waved off. On another try, it waved off again.

"At this point we'd been laying as many rounds down range as we could, and had been in the fight for a couple of hours," Christian said. "We were about to run out of ammo."

He called in for the chopper again, but was told it would land south of the city, about 500 yards from their position.

Christian and the Marines couldn't believe it. They were out of energy, low on ammunition, and had nothing left to give. So Christian made what he would later call a "rash decision."

"I told one of the young Marines to carry my gun. I picked up the casualty and started running," Christian said. "I didn't give them direction on what I was doing. I just expected them all to understand."

They did. They covered him, and followed. Despite the maze of city streets, Christian knew one alley ran straight down the middle. And that's what he hit, sprinting toward the landing site.

"I ran until I couldn't run anymore," he said. "My legs were on fire, but I kept saying, 'I got you, buddy. I got you.'"

When he was close, he dropped to his knees, winded. The helicopter came down, and other Marines lifted Levy aboard.

He didn't make it. A few days later, in Germany, his mother would make the decision to take the badly wounded Marine off of life support. Christian would be awarded a Silver Star for trying to save Levy's life. To this day,

Levy's mother and Lyn talk on the telephone every week, and see each other as much as possible, their bonds sealed by heroism and heartbreak.

But that was later. First, Christian would face his own struggle for survival.

During that emotionally draining call, Lyn learned the extent of her son's injuries: both of his legs were gone, one from right below his hip, and the other at the knee. His pelvis had imploded, and part of his right index finger was blown off. His left hand and arm were also badly damaged.

In what seemed like an interminable length of time between telephone calls, Christian was being whisked from the battlefield to a triage unit in Afghanistan, then to Landstuhl in Germany.

There doctors make the call when the wounded should be shipped to the States for further care. Christian wasn't ready for such a move. One minute his condition was stable, the next he was in crisis. He was running fevers of 104–105°F. His heart rate and blood pressure would plunge to dangerous levels.

Christian was unaware of all of this. Because of the severity of his injuries he had been slipped into a medically induced coma. "It was too traumatic for him to be awake," Lyn said. Lyn, however, was just beginning to learn how bad things really were. The grave danger her son was in had also led to another decision by the medical team: bring the family over, now!

Lyn received the call to head to Germany and was made aware that his injuries were serious.

What she wasn't told was that doctors feared Christian wasn't going to survive.

"Basically, they tell you that, 'He's here, we're going to let the doctors evaluate him, and they'll tell you what we need to do next,' " Lyn recalls. "Until you're face-to-face, you don't know how bad it is."

In the rush to get to Europe, amid fears for Christian's safety and dreading that he was all alone, Lyn reached out to friends and family in their hometown of Munford, Tennessee. The secretary from Christian's church responded almost immediately, letting the family know that, by chance, one of their members was stationed in Germany. Lyn didn't know the woman, but the church was going to contact her and tell her about Christian. The response was swift and heartwarming. The woman found someone to watch her own children and promised to sit with Christian until his family arrived.

She would be relieved at times by one of Christian's fellow Marines, a friend who once was a roommate but was now stationed in Germany.

"That was such a relief to me," Lyn said. "It made me feel really good to know he wasn't alone."

During a time of such uncertainty for Lyn and her family, having the woman and a Marine there for Christian was comforting, and a sign of hope. They were being watched over.

"There were two miracles right off the bat," she thought. "What were the odds that would happen?"

Finally, on December 16, Lyn saw her son. He was still in a coma, and would be kept that way for almost one month. He'd had at least four major surgeries by then, and there would be many more. His pelvis had been patched together. His right leg had only three inches of femur left. The left had been lost midway through the knee—and eventually doctors would remove the rest of the knee. Half of his trigger finger was gone from his right hand, and he was in danger of losing three fingers on the left. There was also tissue damage to his left bicep, from shrapnel, as well as burns up and down the inside of that arm.

"I was so distraught, so upset," Lyn remembers. "It was just overwhelming. I struggled so much, knowing I had encouraged him to pursue a life in the military. I had a lot of guilt."

However, what mattered most was that she was with Christian.

"I just never left his side," she said with conviction. "Straight from Germany to Walter Reed in Bethesda. There is no way that anyone could keep me from being with my son."

When Christian first arrived at Walter Reed, Lyn's ex-husband, David, was with her, though he eventually had to return to work. One of Christian's uncles, Richard, stayed longer, but he too would have to get back to his life in South Carolina.

Lyn would stay. This was her new life.

"I wasn't leaving," Lyn said, calmly, the firmness unmistakable through her Southern accent. "No way in hell." No one who knew her should have been surprised. In fact, she'd come to Christian's rescue at another pivotal point in his life, two decades ago.

He was born in Mississippi, to Lyn's sister, Lou.

"His mom wasn't ready to take care of him," says Lyn, a tall brunette with sparkling brown eyes. "She had addiction problems, and would go back and forth with them. She'd get hold of it and then lose control again. We tried to give her every opportunity we could to straighten out, but she lost in the end. We thought it would be best if Christian came over to be with us, where he was safe, and where he'd have the best possible chance of a normal existence.

"I've had Chris since he was four years old. He's as much my son as any of my other children."

The Reed clan includes Christian's brother Justin, whom Lyn also took in shortly after he was born, as well as Nathan, twenty-nine; Corina, twenty-five; and their youngest son, Bobby, twenty-two. The baby of the family is Madison, ten, who was just seven when Christian was wounded. She visits her mother and Christian in Washington during the summers and school breaks, keeping herself busy reading books, finding other kids to play with, and helping Christian in whatever way she can. This bright-eyed, gifted young girl has had to grow up more quickly than her friends back home in Munford.

Though Lyn comes from a military family—her father is a retired Navy commander—only Christian ever expressed an interest in joining the service. It was an idea that came and went in the years after high school, as he bounced from one job to another. There were girlfriends he was reluctant to leave, but he was also exploring other career possibilities. The young man who would become a Marine even entered the seminary for a time, the Brownsville Revival School of Ministry in Pensacola, Florida. When his pastor there started a seminary in Tennessee, Christian returned home to attend. But the old calling to the military proved to be a stronger pull.

"He made the decision and came home one day and said, 'Guess what? I joined the Marine Corps,'" Lyn recalls.

"Ever since I was little my idea of a good time was to go to the Army Surplus store, get canteens and belts, and go out in the woods, playing Army, Marines, whatever you want to call it," Christian said. Having two grandfathers who served was also influential, as were the terrorist attacks in 2001.

"9/11 hit me to the core, like it did every American," Christian said. "I felt a sense of pride to join and know I'd contribute to making sure something like that never happened again."

"I was glad he did it," Lyn said. "It was what he'd wanted all along, though he'd let other things steer him in different directions. I thought it was a good decision, though he joined during wartime and I wasn't crazy about him being on the front lines. Of course it was scary. Every mom is going to be scared. So I was proud and scared at the same time."

Christian left for boot camp on April 13, 2009, and his family was with him in Parris Island, South Carolina, when he graduated that July. After a month's leave, he was off to infantry school, where he learned he'd soon deploy to Afghanistan.

"So it was bam, bam, bam, with no in-between time," Lyn said.

He went overseas right before Christmas, December, 15, 2009.

"I was scared to death," Lyn added. "You didn't know what to think about communications, how to keep in contact or anything like that."

She was surprised when he was able to keep in touch by satellite phone during the seven months he was deployed near Marjah in Helmand Province. Upon his return, Christian had a year stateside, and then was sent back to Afghanistan, this time to Sangin and Kajaki.

"The second deployment was a different story," Lyn said. "We hardly ever heard from him. He was in a bad place and was busy every day. I'm sure someone had a satellite phone, but he had no time to use it."

Christian said the second deployment was far more intense than the first: "Things had ramped up so much kinetically; we couldn't take our eyes off the target. Between that and people being taken out, we didn't want to call home. We were just trying to keep our emotions in check, forget everything, and make it through tomorrow."

For Lyn, it was a different life, being part of a military family again. She and her sister and brother had grown up in that environment, traveling the world with their mom and dad. But it wasn't what Lyn chose when it came time to raise her family. They settled in Tennessee. There, in Munford, a small town 25 miles north of Memphis, Lyn raised her family and had a longtime job as a pharmacy technician. She'd never considered leaving for any length of time—until that 6:00 a.m. phone call. Suddenly, the quiet family life in Tennessee was no longer an option, at least as far as Lyn was concerned.

Though she was determined to stay and be with Christian, it was a difficult decision for all concerned. Despite the best of intentions, there are tensions and stress that accompany attempts to maintain a long-distance marriage. Her husband, Lyn said, sometimes felt she was spending too much time away from home. Her company kept her on medical leave as long as they could, but when they were bought out by a bigger firm, her position was eliminated. And being on call 24-7 for one child in a hospital far from home meant not being there for the other people she cared about most in her life.

"It's hard because your whole life and family are 863 miles away," Lyn said. "And life goes on there day-to-day regular, while you're dealing with things up here. You're missing the rest of the family, and they're missing you, and you do things they don't experience." At times she wishes her life were different, that she could wake up from the nightmare that began with an explosion in Afghanistan.

"My daughter was seven when this all happened, and she's had two birthdays without me, in May. I wasn't home either time. . . . I feel like I've missed out on a whole big chunk of her life. But at the same time, I wouldn't dare leave Christian on his own either. It's hard to just leave and basically start a new life. But somebody has to do it."

That new life began in Germany.

With her son still in a coma, Lyn had two immediate worries that kept her glued to his bedside. First, of course, was whether he would even be able to survive. Second, if he woke up, even for a second, she wanted to be right there. In the meantime, while he was unconscious, she was going to make Christian know he was loved and supported by touching him and talking to him. "I still believe they can hear you, even when they are in a coma," Lyn said.

Christian's condition remained questionable, but doctors wanted to get him to Walter Reed as soon as possible. On the afternoon of December 19, just six days after he had been blown up, he was on a plane headed home. Any joy for Lyn at this development was overshadowed by Christian's condition on the flight.

"He almost didn't make it over here," Lyn said. "His fever spiked to 105. In all honestly, I wish they'd kept him in Germany and got him more stable before he made the trip."

Arriving stateside meant more of the same, as Christian struggled with fevers, infections, and a weak heartbeat.

"The worst day was Christmas Day," Lyn explained. "He almost died on Christmas. His heart would go down to ten beats per minute, and then come back up. He spiked fevers that would not go down. He had to be kept in a cooling vest to keep his temperature under control. It was a frightening thing to witness."

Christian spent the first month in intensive care, and then doctors thought he was stable enough to go out on the floor. Lyn didn't agree, especially because he was still on a ventilator and needed to be suctioned. Someone needed to keep a constant eye on him, she thought.

"In the ICU, you have a full-time nurse assigned to you," Lyn said. "On the floor, you share a nurse with other patients."

He was soon back in the ICU, with gallbladder problems. It needed to be removed, but doctors weren't sure Christian was strong enough for another major procedure, Lyn remembers. Instead, they installed a drain and put him on massive doses of antibiotics, and his condition slowly improved.

Waking up from the coma was a gradual process. When the doctors first decreased his medication, Christian didn't respond. "He wasn't waking up and we were getting really concerned," Lyn said. This was only a month since the blast, and his heart rate was still alarmingly erratic. "We were still concerned that he wasn't going to make it," Lyn recalls.

He was awake enough on January 11 to receive his Purple Heart from the commandant of the Marine Corps. "These young guys are on so much medication as a result of their horrendous injuries, that they are kind of in a medication fog for quite a long time," Lyn said. "He made sure he had a haircut, his first shave, and his cammies blouse on for the pinning of the Purple Heart, and the pinning of his recent meritorious promotion to Corporal, dated December 2."

When he was finally awake, though still groggy, Christian learned that no other Marine had been hurt in the blast that wounded him. This was his major concern. Only after knowing his buddies were okay did Christian begin to face the extent of his own injuries.

"There was no preparation," Christian said. "I looked down one day—I knew I'd have to—I looked down and realized the rest of me wasn't there. Fuck.

"That was my reaction. 'Fuck.' "

At that time, Christian was also beginning to recognize people and could respond to simple commands.

"Finally, a little bit more and a little bit more, he started to wake, but he didn't know what was going on," Lyn said. "Another week would go by and he was more alert, and more able to ask a question or two. We'd try to tell him he was in Bethesda, but the whole time he was on a ventilator with this large tube in his neck—so he couldn't communicate."

An enterprising nurse suggested a magnet board with letters for him to use, so Lyn bought one at a nearby Toys "R" Us. But even that presented its own set of problems. His right arm was bandaged because of the amputations, his left because of skin grafts. Moving the letters was difficult and time-consuming. It took more than an hour to spell out one part of his first request—a pickle. He also wanted a Dr. Pepper. His family was thrilled that he was communicating, but both requests were denied.

It was Lyn who noticed what she now refers to as Christian's "Elvis snarl." The move involved a slight curl of his lip that Christian didn't even know he was doing. Nevertheless, it provided endless amusement for his family. When they finally described it to him, he would "snarl" on command.

Such moments helped the family believe that they had Christian back. He was going to live.

"Going back to the ICU for the gallbladder surgery was really scary," Lyn said, "but we started to be warily confident that he was going to be all right.

"After five months as an inpatient, or an 'impatient' as we joked, Christian was on the road to recovery," said Lyn. The next milestone Christian achieved was being healthy enough to be discharged to outpatient status. Christian and Lyn would move to Building 62—into a two-bedroom apartment where he could convalesce and receive physical therapy across the street.

But even that minor cause for celebration came with complications. They also learned then that Christian had cardiomyopathy. Until then, the family thought his heart problems were medication-related. Now, it seemed, the trauma of the last six months may have permanently weakened his heart. It was another treatment to undergo, another hurdle in an endless battle off the battlefield.

"We learned that his heart was only pumping at 35 percent efficiency," Lyn said. "We were scared all over again. It's just one more thing he'll have to deal with for the rest of his life. That being said, the care Christian received from the time of the blast to now has been incredible. Without the expert care of the military medical system, I know Chris wouldn't be here with us today. For that I am eternally grateful. We have formed lifelong relationships with certain nurses and corpsmen that took excellent care of Christian. We all have our 'favorites,' and you know who you are. Corpsmen who sat with us all night if needed, and nurses who wore gloves on their heads to make you laugh when they would come in our room just to brighten your day."

The move to Building 62 didn't just change Christian's status, and both of their living arrangements. (Lyn had spent the past six months living at the Navy Lodge.) The change also meant Lyn officially became her son's non-medical attendant (NMA), essentially his private nurse, executive assistant, scheduler, chauffeur, cheerleader, cleaning service, and more. Of course she'd been doing many of these tasks already, but now she had a Department of Defense title and a stipend. (The military provides part of the stipend directly to the caregiver and part through the wounded warrior to help ensure that the service member has input into his care.)

In essence, the move confirmed the reality: Lyn was Christian's full-time caregiver. "Now I provide the care that the hospital was providing before," Lyn said. "Wound care and the things that help his day-to-day living, like preparing meals, getting laundry done, and keeping up the apartment, are just a few of the things that I do for Chris on a daily basis. What most people don't realize is that, for these guys, even doing a simple thing like cleaning the shower, or doing laundry, can be a painful and even dangerous task. As a mom and a caregiver, I am with him 24-7 and can see when he needs help. And, because I am his mom, he isn't embarrassed or afraid to ask me for help."

A major aspect of the job is arranging the cornucopia of daily medicines, seeing that he takes them all, and, equally important, making sure he doesn't run out.

"The biggest part is making sure they're safe," Lyn said of the work she and other Walter Reed moms do. "They are double, triple, or quadruple amputees, who are at extreme risk all the time. There are wounds that need to be dressed and watched, delicate skin that has to heal, and therapy sessions that have to be attended. All of these items need to be cared for and will never go away."

There is no "official" training for Lyn and other family support members, though without them, their sons and daughters would face a longer and less productive recovery. That hit home for Lyn when Christian was first transferred out of the ICU.

"That transition from the ICU to the fourth floor was the scariest part for me," she said. "I was given more responsibility, essentially becoming a caregiver on a twenty-four-hour basis, along with my brother's help."

When Christian started throwing up at one point, she desperately tried to keep it from going down his tracheostomy tube. "I did a lot of button-pushing to get the nurses in there right away," Lyn said. "But you learn very quickly when it's a life-and-death situation, and you have to know what to do."

After spending so many months in the hospital, most of the Mighty Moms caught on quickly when it came to the care their sons and daughter required. Lyn learned how to redress Christian's wounds on weekends when the wound-care team was off duty, among so many other caregiver tasks. Common sense and concern for a loved one also come in handy. Lyn decided early on, for example, to take care of things when Christian needed to go to the bathroom. Knowing that he was too proud to ask for a stranger's help—and too impatient to wait for it—she would step in without being asked.

These are not the roles that Lyn and Christian imagined for themselves, but they made it work.

"What twenty-nine-year-old wants to live with his mom?" Lyn asks, laughing. "He knows I'm there to help him, and we do the best we can with the situation. He gets on my nerves and I get on his, and we have our tiffs, but then we move on."

Eighteen months after he was critically wounded, Christian is more independent. He can come and go more as he pleases. He's driving. He's been hunting and fishing, around the Washington area and back home in Tennessee. But he's almost never on his own.

"We try to give him as much independence as possible," Lyn said. "He needs help to get into the boat and things like that, so he's never really alone for any length of time, just the drive from here to there."

Similarly, the moms of Walter Reed are never really alone either. They are a nonstop sisterhood of the scrubs, supporting their wounded sons and daughters, as well as each other.

"The moms stick together," Lyn said. "We're our own chain of information. The best way to find something out is to find someone who's been there and done it before. And, make no mistake, they are each other's biggest fans.

"When you first get here, the other moms come to you individually and introduce themselves. They tell you, 'If you need help, I'm here.' And that's how we survive. It is beyond belief the amount of information that it takes to not only be a good caregiver, but to take care of yourself. Without the support of all of these wonderful moms here, who are now some of my closest friends, I don't know where I would be. We are from all walks of life, but we share a common bond—the love of our sons. These are some of the bravest and strongest people I know."

As hard as it sometimes is to imagine after such a long run at Walter Reed, Lyn and Christian will one day return to Tennessee—Lyn to her home, and Christian to one that will be built for him, thanks to the Gary Sinise Foundation and the Tunnel to Towers Foundation. He will, eventually, regain more independence, but they are looking for a piece of property for him that is not far from Lyn's. The family wants to ensure that, should she be needed, she's nearby. Christian will always need a certain amount of support, in part to help with his physical disabilities, but also for nonphysical wounds.

One of the "signature wounds" of the wars in Iraq and Afghanistan is traumatic brain injury, or TBI. It's caused in many cases by the trauma that the brain incurs when a soldier or Marine is knocked in the head after an explosion. Though Christian hasn't been diagnosed with a severe case, his mom, who schedules his appointments and keeps track of his medicine, has noticed some changes in his behavior since the injury.

"He had always been a little forgetful," Lyn said, "but it really was worsened by the explosion. His memory is definitely not what it was, but he is participating in therapy sessions to address these issues. A lot of them are dealing with that."

An incident over a July Fourth holiday raised a further worry for Lyn. They were attending a backyard barbecue at the home of a friend in Essex, Maryland. All was well—until the fireworks started. Suddenly, from out of the darkness, Lyn heard Christian screaming her name. She turned and saw that he was petrified and crying uncontrollably.

Lyn and her daughter Madison rushed Christian into the car, leaving behind towels and shoes. She gently patted his shoulder, telling him he was safe and that he would be okay. She reassured him that they were leaving and only then did he seem to calm down.

"It lasted about twenty minutes," Lyn said. "Once he was back in the car and driving home, I said: 'What happened?' He told me, 'The rapid popping of the fireworks sounded like machine-gun fire and I had to get out of there.'"

As he calmed down, about a half hour into their drive home, Lyn could feel herself getting emotional.

"I couldn't control the tears from rolling down my face," Lyn recalled. "I didn't even realize I was crying. I feel bad that he has experiences like that. It's just something that he will have to deal with the rest of his life, but, hopefully, can learn how to control."

Christian and Lyn had attended events with fireworks before, but the displays had been much farther away. Being close up was the trigger in this case, Lyn believes.

"You never know when episodes will happen and he'll get into that dark spell," she said. "You're constantly walking a tightrope on how you think they'll behave that day."

The episode was a reminder to Lyn that the Marine Corps, as well as all branches of the military, need to make counseling for post-traumatic stress disorder mandatory. While counseling is offered to all wounded warriors, it is often the furthest thing from their minds. After all, they are trained to be tough. And the idea of sitting down with a counselor and revealing their innermost thoughts would be tantamount to weakness in their eyes. That's why Christian has not sought help. "What Marine will say, 'I need counseling'?" Lyn asks. His mother has. She says, "I thought if I could get help, I could understand how to help him, because he won't ask for help."

The unexpectedness of the attack over July Fourth has also renewed her conviction that she was needed while Christian stayed at Walter Reed. Lyn said that the military had been considering cutting back on nonmedical attendants, and Lyn was told that she might not be able to remain for the duration of her son's time at Building 62.

"That's another reason I'm insisting I don't need to go home," she said. "These things happen, and what could happen to him if no one's there?"

If her time at Walter Reed has taught Lyn anything, it's how to speak up for her son. "I used to be very shy, but all that's gone. I can honestly say I am not the same person I was before Chris was injured. I am my own person now and I can talk to anybody," Lyn said. "And you have to be their advocate. A lot of times they can't advocate for themselves—or won't.

"These guys deserve everything they can get to physically and mentally heal. They've given everything up in their lives that they can give for their country. The least we can do is make sure things go as they should, without them being taken advantage of or just being forgotten about."

More important than the changes Lyn has seen in herself are the ones she's seen in Christian.

"A year ago he didn't want to live," Lyn said. "He was in a very dark place. He didn't want to live like this. He sat in his room with the shades pulled. He didn't want to go out. He was miserable.

"That was a long time, and it was very hard to watch. I try to encourage him, and get him to do the things he should do, and sometimes you get shot down. You're scared to death that he would do something to himself. I don't think he would, but it's always a question in the back of my mind."

A trip home to Tennessee seemed to make all the difference for Christian.

In September 2012, he went home for a high school football benefit. He learned, Lyn said, that "his friends were still his friends. They didn't care if he had legs or not. He was still Chris. He didn't get that until he went home and actually saw it."

When he went hunting, Christian's dad wanted to stay with him, but Christian sent him off to his own tree stand. He needed to do it himself.

"It's easier to learn when someone isn't sitting over you, staring, or asking, 'Can I help you?'" Christian says. "Instead of having that, you're forced to learn things the way you need to learn them—without having help, or the looks, or worrying about what people think.

"You just want to feel as normal as possible. You want to feel, 'It's fucking unfortunate but I'm not incapable,' you know what I mean?" Christian added.

He returned to Tennessee a few months later, and hunted every day. "People still treated him the same," Lyn said, "and he was still able to do what he loves to do. That's when he found the desire to live."

Christian said, "It definitely took a long time to get there. A lot of it was getting the medication right, and making the pain go away."

He hopes to share what he found at home with other service members and veterans, and has begun a nonprofit called Gunslinger Outfitters, which takes wounded warriors and other veterans out on guided hunts and fishing outings. If there is something they want to do, he's willing to help them figure it out. And he's setting a good example.

"A month ago I was on a jet ski wide open, with no legs," Christian says. "It was hilarious. People couldn't believe it."

Christian's epiphany has helped his mom too. "I feel somewhat at ease. He's doing things that make him happy and is in a much better place," Lyn said. "My days are a whole lot easier than they were."

But there were those days that weren't easy, moments that she was determined that Christian not see.

"If I'm having a moment, and getting ready to cry, I do it while he's not around, or leave the room," Lyn said. "I don't want him to see it's affecting my life, or give him guilt he doesn't need to deal with." It was a rule she made others follow as well. "I used to tell people, 'If you're going to cry, you can stay outside. Come in here with a happy game face. You can't let him see you upset because that will upset him.' "

What also got her through those moments since that 6:00 a.m. phone call was faith.

"If I didn't have that, I don't know what I'd do," Lyn said. "I can't say I never asked why. I did. But I kept going back there. I'm a Christian. So is my son. He's struggling with his faith, but is better than when he first came to. God doesn't give us more than we can handle, and everything he does is for a purpose. I am fully sure there is one, and Chris is coming around. Somewhere along the line, some good is going to come out of the bad."

To remind her of that faith, she even got a tattoo on her wrist, something she had sworn she'd never do. It's a Bible verse, Joshua 1:9: "Have I not commanded you? Be strong, and courageous. Do not be afraid; do not be discouraged, for the Lord your God will be with you wherever you go." Lyn said, "Sometimes I just needed a visual along the way to remind me that things were going to be okay. Now, I just look down at my wrist and smile, knowing that God always has control, even if we don't."

FOUR

Tyler Jeffries and Pam Carrigan Britt

KNOCK ON THE DOOR. To MOST PEOPLE THAT IS A SIGN OF GOOD THINGS to come—special deliveries, costumed kids on Halloween, or a visit by a special friend or neighbor. But for military families it can mean something entirely different—something unwelcome and ominous.

With just a couple of taps on the door, or the stinging ring of the doorbell, a casualty notification officer (CNO) delivers to the primary next of kin of service members the dreaded news that no one can ever be prepared to hear. The following is a sample script, taken from the Army's official CNO training guide, for the responsibility that the military considers among its highest priorities and most difficult of duties: "The Secretary of the Army has asked me to express his deep regret that your (relationship; son, Robert or husband, Edward; etc.) (died/was killed in action) in (country/state) on (date). (State the circumstances provided by the Casualty Area Command.) The Secretary extends his deepest sympathy to you and your family in your tragic loss."

Pam Carrigan Britt, the mother of US Army Specialist Tyler Jeffries, knew there was always a possibility she might hear that knock on her door. However, she was totally unprepared for "the call."

"I had no idea they would notify the family of a severely injured son or daughter in a terribly impersonal way—by phone," Pam would say later.

Pam, though originally from Tampa, Florida, is a Concord, North Carolina, girl through and through. Her thick blond hair, gentle hazel eyes, and

65

affable smile endear her to everyone she knows. When she speaks—with a pleasing, mellifluous Southern accent—she exudes intelligence, compassion, and a quality she recently discovered in herself—defiance!

Before the call, Pam was a full-time mom and a logistics coordinator for Jacobson's Logistics, which handles freight for the Food Lion Corporation in Salisbury, North Carolina. Though originally trained as a medical technician—a skill she would eventually be thankful for—she managed the inbound freight that the chain of grocery stores received on a daily basis.

After graduating from high school, Tyler worked at a few different jobs, but wanted something more fulfilling. He decided to enlist in the US Army, but had to delay his basic training because there was such a long waiting list. Tyler wanted to be in the infantry, and couldn't wait to experience Army life. In April 2010, this independent young man left for boot camp determined to rid the world of bad guys.

"Tyler just lived for baseball," Pam said. "He loved it, and his dream was to play professionally someday, but it just didn't happen that way. He decided to join the Army, and here we are today."

Pam, though divorced from Tyler's father, has a good relationship with her ex-husband. "We all get along great," Pam said, "and Tyler is close to him as well as my current husband.

"My son has a heart of gold, even though he may not look that way. He is a big, tough guy with broad shoulders and dirty blond hair, and I guess you could say that he is headstrong and very independent," Pam said. "To be honest, I never wanted him to go into the Army, because I knew he would go to Afghanistan. But, considering he is headstrong and a person who wants to do things his way, I knew I had to back off and accept his decision."

Pam, though apprehensive, was still a proud mom, and gave him credit for taking the initiative. "Tyler is a person with extreme determination, and once I accepted the reality of him going to war, I always knew he would come home, or never come home at all," explained Pam. She hadn't heard much about soldiers and Marines coming home wounded. "You hear about the ones who died in the wars, but not as much about those who came home injured. I am aware of the knock on the door the Army uses to notify families that their son or daughter died in the line of duty. But I had no idea they would notify the family of a severely injured son or daughter in a terribly impersonal way—by phone," Pam said, wiping a stream of tears from her cheeks.

But the phone did ring, on Saturday, October 6, 2012. "I was in bed, and a call came in at 5:29 a.m., and I said, 'Is this a joke?' This is the last thing that I expected." In a very matter-of-fact tone, the casualty assistance officer said: "Ma'am, your son has been injured. He sustained a bilateral amputation of both legs after he stepped on an IED while on patrol in southern Afghanistan." The officer read through the medical report, and all Pam could do was cry. She shed tears of joy that Tyler was still alive, but tears of heartbreak that the unthinkable trauma of war had happened to her son.

She later found out the gruesome details. Tyler was on patrol in a village just outside of Kandahar. They were about to leave on a mission when the soldier who was supposed to sweep for mines said he wasn't going to go, believing they had no business being there in the first place, according to Tyler's recollection of events. Tyler volunteered to take the minesweeper, and together, he and his buddies were able to clear most of the village. As they sat down to take a quick break, Tyler's lieutenant said, "Let's get this done," and Tyler replied, "Sure, let's go."

Tyler stood up, and after taking only three steps, a remote-controlled IED exploded under his feet. He never saw it coming.

So many service members who have been blown up by these deadly and deceptive devices in Iraq and Afghanistan don't remember much about the blast. Tyler was the exception. He remembered everything. While he was disoriented for a couple of seconds, he was jarred into consciousness by everybody around him shouting. "He couldn't figure out what was going on, but heard all of his buddies continuing to loudly call his name. He finally yelled back and said: 'What do you want?' As he tried to get up he realized there was something really, really wrong with him," Pam said.

Since his patrol was in a remote area, it took the medevac helicopter almost an hour to reach him. He lessened his anxiety by laughing and cracking jokes with his buddies, who by that point had put three tourniquets on each leg, and were keeping him awake and engaged—all part of their military training for cases just like this.

The man on the phone gave Pam more bad news. Tyler had severe burns on his arms and nose. He lost his right leg below the knee, and his left leg at the knee, though it was unclear if that knee could be saved.

Hearing the extent of his injuries, Pam immediately thought of Tyler's other reason for enlisting. "You know, Tyler had a three-year-old daughter, and I had my concerns with that," Pam said. "Her name is Ella, and she was born in September 2010. Tyler was considering a military career when he found out his girlfriend was pregnant. He decided to join the Army because he wanted to make sure both mother and child were taken care of financially, and would not have to worry about money.

"During the time he was under medical care, I knew his burns would heal, and he would be walking someday on prosthetic legs. I also knew he may never be able to have children again due to the injuries he sustained. It was a comfort for me to know that he had this beautiful child; that was the reason she's here," Pam said.

In one conversation before he enlisted, Tyler told his mom that if he ever lost his legs in the war he wouldn't want to live. After the call, her thoughts were racing. He just lost both of his legs. Would he be suicidal? Would he lose the will to live? She dropped to the floor and wept, but knew she couldn't fall apart for too long. Tyler needed her.

Four hours later, the phone rang again. "Hi, Mom; it's me. You know I lost my legs."

"I know, honey," Pam said, trying to hold back tears and keep calm for Tyler.

"Mom, I don't want you to worry," Tyler said. "I'll be okay."

As all parents of severely wounded warriors know, the most difficult time is between receiving the call and arriving at the hospital. Their children aren't right there to comfort, there are a million things to prepare, and all their worst fears are magnified a hundredfold. Pam knew that Tyler's flight would arrive in the US on Tuesday, and there were so many things she had to organize before she left.

"This was an incredibly stressful time in my life," Pam said, "and what made it even worse was that I had worked for Food Lion only ninety days, and had no idea if I would have a job when I came back."

With her life in complete chaos, Pam nevertheless decided to talk to her boss in person and take things from her desk that she thought she could use during what she knew would be a long stay in Bethesda. "As soon as I got the call about Tyler I contacted my boss and told her what happened and that I didn't know when I would be back. My life was in complete disarray, and I kept thinking I would lose my house, my husband, my job, my life—everything." Pam was on mental and physical overdrive.

Though expecting the worse, Pam was comforted by the empathy and concern her boss showed, and she was surprised that her boss followed up with a call only an hour later. "My boss couldn't have been more wonderful. She told me that they talked and didn't want to lose me and that my fellow employees—many of whom I never met—donated their time off so that I could take my time off with pay. She told me to take whatever time I needed, and my job would be waiting for me when I got back. I was relieved that she would consider this as just a leave of absence, and she reiterated that when I got settled she would talk to me about working remotely."

Sadly, this is not always the case. The employers of other moms of severely wounded warriors were sympathetic at first, but over time they fired them, sometimes in one of the most heartless ways possible—by email.

Pam, her husband, her father, her son and her son's wife, and their ten-month-old grandson were getting ready to see Tyler for the first time. On Monday, after she emptied her desk at work, she and her family headed, in separate cars, to Walter Reed, where Tyler would be treated after being stabilized overseas. During the grueling seven-hour trek, her emotions were on steroids. Nothing could have prepared her for this moment of truth. She knew she would be tested as a mom, and a human being. Would she be ready?

After what seemed like an eternity, she finally arrived at Walter Reed, overwhelmed by the sheer size and scope of the base.

"My heart was pounding—I had no idea where to go. As I was driving toward the parking lot, which was called the America Garage, I felt completely frightened and alone," Pam said. "Once I parked my car I just started to cry hysterically. I suddenly realized there was no one there to help me get to where I needed to go." Then she remembered she had the phone number of another mom, Maureen Crabbe, whose son was also blown up by an IED, and was being treated at the hospital. Pam had gotten Maureen's contact information from another Mighty Mom, Siobhan Fuller-McConnell, whom she met on Facebook and whose son, Derek, had also been a patient at Walter Reed.

"I was lucky to have Maureen's number programmed in my phone, and I called her as soon as I found it. Thank goodness she answered right away, and was there on campus to meet me," Pam said.

As she waited anxiously for Maureen to arrive, she couldn't hold back her tears, and when Maureen finally did find Pam, she just fell into her arms, limp as a rag doll. As only a mom in a similar situation could instinctively do, Maureen held Pam close and felt her pain in silence. After a few minutes she tried to comfort Pam, assuring her that everything would be okay, and led her across the street to Building 62 and then eventually to the hospital.

The two made their way through the long hospital hallways; they were deeply pained to see so many wounded young men and women. Some had both legs cut above the knees, some below; others were missing arms and legs, and more had burns on their faces and other parts of their bodies. Some were inpatients; others were returning to the hospital for their rehabilitation sessions.

The reality of the situation struck Pam at her core. Tyler, her independent, headstrong, and determined young son, was now a wounded warrior. It was an incredible burden for her to bear. Pam just wanted to see Tyler and make sure that no matter what was missing or intact, she could hold him and tell him everything was going to be okay.

Pam and her family waited about four hours for Tyler's flight to arrive, and for him to be transported to Walter Reed, where he immediately was taken to the ICU. "When I finally got to the third floor where Tyler was being treated, instinct just kicked in," said Pam. "I hugged him and kissed him, and I was just so happy that he was alive. Though he was heavily sedated, I know he was glad that I was there, too, though I could see on his face that he was a little down and afraid. He said: 'Mom, you know I won't be able to ride a roller coaster ever again,' and I told him that there are many other things in life you will be able to do; let's just think about those other things."

Fortunately for Pam, her sister is a registered nurse. She arrived at the hospital the next day, as did many family members and close friends and relatives, and helped Pam understand the medical issues she was facing. Tyler was heavily medicated, which is typical immediately after receiving a catastrophic wound. "It was so difficult to see your own son in a state like that. He would wake up and was extremely disoriented, and would ask, 'Where am I?' I guess he could see my anxiety because he would often tell me not to worry, that everything was going to be okay. The doctors were very good in explaining what was happening to Tyler medically, and I knew what to expect. The most important thing to me was that Tyler never wakes up and has me not be there." For Pam, who had been looking forward to welcoming home her healthy young soldier someday, her dream was forever shattered.

While Pam had hoped that the first time she'd see Tyler back in America would not be in a hospital, as far as hospitals go, Walter Reed is exceptional.

The physical facility is clean and easily accessible, the medical staff competent and caring, and there is no shortage of well-meaning volunteers who want to help wounded warriors. It's just not where Pam wanted to be, and certainly not where she wanted to see Tyler.

"In my early career I was a medical assistant, though I haven't worked in that field for years," she said. However, even with that background, as Pam began to settle in to her new reality, as well as her new temporary residence in the Fisher House, a nonprofit organization that provides free housing for families of wounded warriors, she realized she had a lot to learn. Tyler's wounds were severe. He had to have 170 stitches near his pelvis, and a dressing that had to be changed three or four times a day, as well as dressings on his two stumps. To make matters worse, he had to endure a urinary catheter for six weeks, which he received in the field the day of the injury. Unfortunately, it perforated his urethra nine times, which resulted in a complete reconstruction.

"It amazes me now, looking back, how much I had to learn in such a short time—like learning how to care for wounds. It's kind of trial and error, and I learned it by spending weeks and weeks in the hospital room," said Pam. While the nursing staff was good about changing Tyler's dressings and responding to her need for help, she also began to see that they had other patients who needed their attention, and Tyler was often uncomfortable with the nurses coming in and out of his room. Pam explains how she learned to advocate for Tyler: "I would go to the nurses' station and say, 'I know you are busy, but can you give me the supplies and I'll do it myself?' They didn't always like it, but I certainly wasn't going to let my son die!"

It was tough for Tyler, too. Aside from his physical injuries, he had to deal with many doctors, nurses, and residents constantly coming in, and there were days he just wanted to be left alone. Pam knew Walter Reed was a teaching hospital, and the throngs of medical professionals visiting day after day would only improve the care for all of the patients. Still, she was devoted to her new role as medical advocate, full-time nurse, psychologist, and most of all, a dynamic and at times defiant Mighty Mom.

Tyler was clearly happy to have his mom by his side. There were times, though, that he was between a rock and a hard place. He didn't want his mom changing his dressings, but it was even more uncomfortable having a "hot" twenty-five-year-old nurse do it. "Tyler would at first say that he didn't want me to change his dressings, but he finally said he would rather have his mom help than the young nurses. He would joke with the nurses, telling them, 'You don't have to do that for me, my mom will take care of that.' " Pam knew that even though Tyler was handling the situation so bravely and courageously, deep down he was afraid. He would often confide in her that he was worried about his future, if anyone would ever love him, and if he would be the same person he was before the injury. And who wouldn't be? This strong, young soldier, who could carry a pack that weighed more than one hundred pounds, survive on little food and sleep, and still be able to perform with top-gun precision, now needed his mom to take care of his every need.

"There was one day when at least a dozen rather insensitive medical people came in to Tyler's room, pulling off all of his covers without any regard for his modesty. It was very embarrassing for him. I just had to say, 'Wait a minute. Can you give my son some privacy?' I guess it was then that I realized that I would never leave his side. Not for one second, unless there was someone I trusted there to take my place." Despite his internal soldier, Tyler still needed to feel the comfort and protection of his mom.

As the weeks went by, Tyler's wounds were healing well, so well in fact that he was scheduled to be fitted for prosthetic legs after only a couple of months in the hospital. But he still struggled with gaining the confidence he needed to do the things he did before, and come to grips with his new life reality.

"For me, it took quite a while until I could process what actually happened," Pam said. "I was torn between still wanting to take care of my responsibilities at home and my injured child. And it was very hard watching him struggle with doing everyday things that were second nature before the blast. I feel like a horrible person sometimes, too, because I don't get back to people as much as I should, and I feel so emotionally drained and overwhelmed every day. But I am inspired by my son, too. He refuses to throw himself a 'pity party,' and the Army did teach him to be positive and self-reliant."

Pam credits his speedy recovery to many things: comprehensive medical and nursing care, a supportive group of family and friends, and the other devoted moms of wounded warriors. "I am fortunate that I have a great family and a wonderful, supportive husband, but I can tell you this has ried my marriage," Pam said. "It's hard to be away from your family and your husband for so long. My husband has been wonderful through this entire ordeal, but at the end of the long stressful days at the hospital, many days I just did not have anything left in me to give to anyone else. Emotionally I was just drained, and my husband was 400 miles away at home, and longing for any updates or news of Tyler's progress. I struggled to open up and talk. Sometimes I just wanted to shut the world out, and pretend that if I didn't talk about it, then I would wake up from the bad dream I was living."

But the Mighty Moms are always there for each other. They are as close as if they were all friends for years, sharing their own war stories in an effort to keep each other out of harm's way. "One of the first things a Marine mom told me was to keep a journal, and write down everything. And thank God I did."

Mothers' bonds with their children are undeniable.

They feel their pain, relish their accomplishments, and look forward to them having young ones of their own. They are the first line of defense against bullies, recalcitrant teachers, colds and sore throats, and a myriad of real and perceived enemies during childhood. They share their lives with other moms on the soccer field, at PTA meetings, and during lunch breaks at work. But as they arrive at Walter Reed to support sons and daughters who have lost limbs, or suffered traumatic brain injuries, or burns and internal wounds, these moms join an exclusive club, a members-only organization that exists simply to assuage the horrors of war.

When Pam settled in to her new home away from home at Walter Reed, she began to accept her new reality, though it continued to feel like a surreal experience. Tyler had been in the hospital for four months, and was soon to become an outpatient. While she would never want an experience like this again, still, there were many heartwarming moments. Like the time she got a call from the front gate telling her that the regional manager from Food Lion was there with five big bags of groceries for her and Tyler. Or, when she met Food Network Chef Robert Irvine, one of her idols, at the "Invincible Spirit Festival" that actor Gary Sinise and his foundation host at the base each year. Above all, it was the other moms who gave her strength, helped her heal, and provided relief from the awful existence that they alone know.

"One of the wives of another wounded warrior who was at Walter Reed with us said to me one day, 'Pam, you know I think that all of you moms are much stronger than any of us wives.' I don't consider myself stronger than a spouse at all. My real strength is at home, but since I've been here, the other moms really help. I wouldn't have gotten through this for the past ten months if not for them."

Wives of the young soldiers and Marines who are treated at Walter Reed are the legal decision makers when their spouses are injured. They can also live with them when they are rehabilitating, and, of course, have power of attorney should the wounded warrior become incapacitated.

But, for the moms, things work a bit differently. While they can and do live with their children on campus, as well as in transitional housing such as the apartments and emergency services that the nonprofit Operation Homefront provides, their financial and legal arrangements can be more complicated.

They are considered NMA's (nonmedical attendants) and are paid a nominal amount—$72 a day—to provide care for their children 24-7. The moms who are married can rely on their spouses at home for financial and emotional support, that is, unless their marriages fall apart from the strain of the calamity. And, sadly, that has happened. "There is not as much support here for the moms as there is for the wives," said Pam, who has formed extremely close relationships with the moms who are in her same situation. "I think it's hard for the people to understand what it is like to be a mom and watch your child suffer every day. But the other moms here know the struggles we are going through with the military, and we all learn through our collective experiences. If I didn't have the other moms around to support me, I would have literally had no one."

Pam added that there are turf issues at Walter Reed just like there are in any organization. "There are wives who have their own support, and moms who have their own groups too, which makes sense since we are all in different stages of life," Pam said.

Thanks to social media such as Facebook and Twitter, Pam was able to connect with moms of other wounded warriors and get advice from them on so many issues that they would otherwise have to learn by default.

Some of the things Pam has learned from the other moms include: be your child's advocate; don't take information at face value; keep copious notes in a daily journal; understand the chain of command; insist your child receives the best care; stand up for your child; communicate with your military liaison; and most of all, take some time for yourself.

"When I first got here I thought I really didn't need anybody," said Pam. "I couldn't have been more wrong! Another thing I learned from the other moms is to not just accept what others are saying. Sometimes you need to speak up and express your concerns. It's the old squeaky wheel theory. But, when your child is helpless and in pain, there is no time to waste, and being passive is simply not an option."

Fortunately, there are volunteers who supplement the social events for this group of strong and dedicated women. Operation Ward 57 hosts cookouts, field trips, and many other activities to take their minds off of their loved ones for a while. Likewise, the Yellow Ribbon Fund provides gift certificates for dinners, as well as for manicures and pedicures; and Luke's Wings helps families fly to many destinations for free, enabling relatives to visit and parents to take a much-needed break. Saks Fifth Avenue in Chevy Chase, Maryland, even gave them a "day of beauty," with free makeovers and sample products from Bobbi Brown, one of the bestselling makeup lines in the country. Irma Murphy, the makeup artist for Bobbi Brown, has a son in high school who is in junior ROTC, and she was thrilled to organize the event. There is no shortage of caring Americans who want to help wounded warriors and their families, and these nonprofit organizations truly help the moms get through the years at Walter Reed.

But the "band of mothers" provides the daily and ongoing support network for each other. "Sometimes we all just get together for dinner and laugh, and talk about how unbelievable our lives are. There are other times that we just hang out and don't really talk about a thing at all. The bottom line for me is that without my built-in group of girlfriends, I don't know how I would have ever gotten through this horrendous experience. We all have a common bond—and that is the absolute love and devotion for our sons and daughters. No mom should ever have to go through this, but if we do, we at least have each other," Pam said.

One of the tragic results of war is the number of US service members who return with injuries—in many cases, catastrophic wounds that troops might not have survived in previous conflicts. As the wars wind down, soldiers like Tyler will be integrated back into the community, and Pam is determined to make sure that his transition is seamless.

"When Tyler and I have been out in public, it is amazing to me how many people just stare," Pam said. "It hurts me so much every time that happens, and I think I will never get over that harsh reality of human behavior. It also amazes me that kids are so much kinder and more understanding than some adults. I have the utmost respect for people who just come up to Tyler and say, 'Thank you for your service.' But, sadly, that always doesn't happen."

One exception is a young autistic boy named Lucas Giese, who has been sending Tyler letters of encouragement and care packages for the past two years. The two have formed a deep bond, and have helped each other tremendously. Tyler even surprised him and his classmates when he showed up at their school for an unexpected visit over the summer.

He also learned to be wary of people who may want to get involved with him just to be in the "limelight," according to Pam. "The fact is that guys like Tyler are considered celebrities, and I am all for that. What Tyler, and all of the soldiers and Marines, have done for our country is something that should be celebrated," Pam added. "On the flip side, these are all good-looking guys who can also be perceived as meal tickets for young girls on the prowl."

Pam has had to learn how to deal with someone with a disability, too. She never thought she might someday have to live with, or take care of, someone with a catastrophic injury like Tyler's. "I would say I'm still learning what to do. This is still so new to me, but I love my child, and want him to have the best life possible. Tyler wants to be a normal person just like the rest of us."

For Pam, one of the toughest issues is helping Tyler realize that he is the same person he was before—lovable, adorable, headstrong, independent, smart, and loyal. "I am continuously amazed by his resilience and resolve," Pam said. The fact that he lost his legs doesn't block him from the possibility of having a great future and living a life of purpose. "I want the world to look at people with disabilities—seen or unseen—no differently than you or me," said Pam. "He may have to adjust to his new life in a different way than the average person, but he isn't the average person, and never was. If every American would look beyond the physical injury and just see the person, well, that would be my hope. And for those who choose to stare, I say they should look at themselves."

Tyler's future is a bright one, and he has dreams of working for a company that builds weapons for the armed forces, near the family's hometown in North Carolina, or opening up his own outdoor shooting range. He is already walking on his prosthetic legs, and every day the process becomes easier. His dream is to go back to school, get his gunsmith degree, and then work full-time. Pam knows her son will succeed in anything he puts his mind to, and is just happy that he is still with her and very much alive. "After this experience I've learned that it is the little things in life that really matter. I look at Tyler and think how fortunate I am to have a son like him, and how his life drama has made me a much stronger person."

This blond Southern gal has become a defiant Mighty Mom.

FIVE

THOMAS MCRAE AND CAROLEE RYAN

T OM MCRAE IS READY TO GO HOME. HE PLANS TO RETIRE TO THE WOODED 10-acre property he owns not far from Camp Lejeune, in North Carolina, his last stateside duty station. There he'll raise his daughter, Aidan, and tend to his horses—he has one now but expects to buy more. And always near, as needed but prepared to give Tom as much room as possible, will be his parents, Carolee and Tim Ryan.

Not everything is in place just yet. The home that is being built for him is still a work in progress. Frankly, so is his recovery. That's not surprising, considering the extent of his injuries. Still, he has made miraculous strides in the two years since he was blown up by an IED while on patrol in the Sangin district of Afghanistan.

Tom, then a staff sergeant and an explosive ordnance disposal (EOD) technician with the US Marine Corps, lost both legs above the knee and his left arm in the blast on January 16, 2012. His right eye was destroyed, and his left was severely damaged. Because of the brain trauma he suffered—bits of shrapnel and bone from around his right eye were blown into his brain—his doctors were initially preparing his family for the worst: "That I may be a one-limbed vegetable forever," as Tom drily puts it today.

Far from it. Speaking to a guest from his motorized wheelchair in the apartment he shares with his family in Building 62 at Walter Reed, he's poised, confident, self-deprecating, and often funny—starting with the olive drab T-shirt he was wearing with the tagline I HAD A BLAST IN AFGHANISTAN blazoned across the back.

He was on track to leave Walter Reed in 2013, but a series of seizures delayed his departure. He needs to go a year without another one before his doctors can sign off on his release—and on his ability to drive, a critical factor for any sense of independence.

"I'm really, really looking forward to getting out of here, out of this area," Tom said. "I don't like the big city. I want to live out in the sticks and collect guns."

While he waits, Tom is making good use of his time. He continues to gain proficiency on his prosthetic legs, and is working on acquiring the four sets he plans to take with him to North Carolina—including short ones for walking around the house, long ones for walking and driving, and a waterproof set so he can tend to his horses in all types of weather. He's also continuing to redevelop the sense of independence he lost since the blast, a loss exacerbated by his traumatic brain injury, by making his way solo around the massive Walter Reed complex to doctors' appointments and physical therapy sessions. At the same time, he's a single father parenting his young daughter.

If he leaves Walter Reed, as hoped, by spring 2014, his "smart home," a house built with the needs of a triple amputee in mind, won't be ready. But knowing that construction is in capable hands—the home is a project of two foundations, Tunnel to Towers and Gary Sinise—Tom is prepared to find something nearby and wait patiently.

"I know for a fact it's not going to be done, so I'll just rent for a little while," Tom said. "It's a temporary situation so it doesn't have to be perfect. It just has to be timely. What's renting for a few months when waiting for your new house to be done?"

Ideal or not, Tom is determined to make a fresh start on his terms, for him, for his daughter, and, at least for the foreseeable future, for the one person who has been by his side almost nonstop since his battered body was brought back to the United States: his mom, Carolee Ryan.

"I plan to move in to the house initially to help him and Aidan out," Carolee said. "And we're looking to buy something close by Tom. There's going to be a transition in general, with him and us: 'Okay, it's time for us to go,' kind of thing. Or maybe mom needs a break, or Tom may need a break."

Whenever the breaks come, they will be well deserved. It's been a long, difficult road since January 2012, one that stretches back all the way to Alaska.

Tom grew up in Juneau, the state capital, where Carolee and her four sisters had been raised by their grandparents. Carolee had three small children—Kristina, age five, Tom, age four, and Rebecca, age three—when Tim came into their lives. She calls Tom a typical Alaska teen growing up. "He liked being outdoors, and hunting and fishing," Carolee said. When, during high school, he started hanging out with what she considered the wrong people, she made a decision crucial to his future, sending him to live with her sister and brother-in-law in Las Vegas. "I knew, as a mom, personally, that he was better, and that there was a better life for him," Carolee said. "We knew that he was worth saving."

It was while in Nevada, during his senior year, that Tom was introduced to the Marine Corps, as recruiters for the various branches of the service set up tables at the high school, passing out flyers and talking to the students. When his parents came down from Alaska for his graduation, they'd learned that he'd already signed up. This was two years before there was a War on Terror, and Carolee was fully supportive of his decision. "I was very proud of him," Carolee said. "I felt that it might give him guidance along the way."

"I thought it would be good for him," Tim agreed, though he pressed the recruiter on why Tom, who had tested well in the screening process, was going into the infantry. "The recruiter said: 'Hey, I tried to talk to him, and get him into a specialized field, but he just wants to jump out of airplanes and helicopters and blow stuff up and shoot machine guns.'"

Tom did become a machine gunner. He was assigned to Twentynine Palms, California, the world's largest Marine Corps base, and attached to Charley Company, 1st Battalion, 7th Marines, a renowned squad that had adopted the nickname "Suicide Charley" after it sustained heavy losses while repelling a much larger Japanese force at Guadalcanal during World War II. After the attack, a flag made of parachute silk and bearing a skull and crossbones, and the words "Suicide Charley," appeared over the position. It's a symbol of endurance and professionalism that members continue to uphold—right down to their Suicide Charley tattoos. It was as part of this modern-day band of brothers that Tom went to Iraq in 2003—the first of his six deployments to the region.

"He was in on the invasion of Iraq," Tim recalled. "He left Kuwait, with a group that secured an oil field in southern Iraq and then proceeded toward Baghdad. He was in on all kinds of stuff. He was in on Fallujah."

During that first deployment, his parents only heard from Tom courtesy of the satellite phone carried by an embedded reporter.

"Three o'clock in the morning, Alaska time, you'd wake up to a call," Tim said. " 'Hi, I'm doing fine. I only have a few seconds on the phone.' "

"And then you'd hear gunfire," Carolee adds, with Tim finishing the thought: "You can hear a firefight going on in the background, and he'd say, 'I gotta go. I gotta go. See ya.' "

After his four-year enlistment was up, Tom left the Corps and returned to Las Vegas, hoping to serve in another capacity, either as a police officer or firefighter. But as the situation deteriorated in Iraq, and the casualties among Marines and soldiers mounted, Tom decided he couldn't sit out the war. When he reenlisted, he was stationed in Hawaii. There, he would marry and apply for one of the military's most dangerous assignments: EOD, a task put in the spotlight because of the prevalence of improvised explosive devices in Iraq and Afghanistan.

"As a mom, you have to be supportive, no matter what, because they're very excited about it," Carolee said. "But it just broke my heart to know he was going to be putting himself in harm's way."

There was at least one practical up side, Tim said: "We thought at the time it was good because he'd be going to school in Florida, and that would keep him out of Iraq and Afghanistan for a little bit, and we could quit watching the news channels."

According to Tim, his son was also thinking long-term. He thought EOD experience would translate well into a civilian job, either with a police force or airport security, after he did twenty years in the Marines.

Aidan was born on April 16, 2008, while Tom was stationed at the Explosive Ordnance School at Eglin Air Force Base in the Florida Panhandle. When he received orders to report to Camp Lejeune later that year, the family moved to North Carolina. Once there, they bought the 10-acre property Tom hopes to return to, but the couple divorced not long after. Tom received primary custody of Aidan; however, she would stay with her mom when he was deployed.

In October 2011, Tom was sent for his second tour in Afghanistan. He'd already done three in Iraq, and had another shipboard deployment to the Mideast. His parents weren't happy, and they provided a rapid-fire tag-team of the concerns they had at the time.

Carolee: "It was a rough deployment for me."

Tim: "Our feelings were that he'd served enough."

Carolee: "This was six deployments. I just remember it being a little bit harder with him being gone, and I didn't know why."

Tim: "She had a premonition something was going to go wrong."

Something did. About a month into the deployment, Tom's friend Dustin Johns, a fellow explosive ordnance tech, lost both legs when an IED detonated. It was Tom who applied the tourniquets that saved Dustin's life.

"When Dustin got injured, I heard from Tom," Carolee said. "He was emotionally upset about it, because they had worked together and he felt extremely . . . I don't know . . ."

"He felt responsible," Tim added.

"He felt responsible for Dustin since he was overseeing him," Carolee agreed. "And so in my heart I thought, 'Well, maybe that's the reason for the anxiety that I was having and we'll make it through this deployment.' "

Despite what she tried telling herself, and the reassurances from others, the worries didn't fade.

"This time was really, really bad," Carolee said. "I don't know why. I think I always worried about him being in Iraq and Afghanistan, but this time was totally different. At work, people said, 'Carolee, he'll make it through,' and I kept saying, 'Okay.' I would try to be strong, I felt like I was being strong, but I just had this gut feeling that it wasn't going to be okay."

Much later, Tom told his dad that this deployment was different for the Marines too.

"There were a lot more IEDs in the time he was there, a lot of them," Tim said. "Tom told me that on that tour he had like, I'm rounding, 130 reports. Now, they file a report every time they disarm a bomb, and he told me that rarely in those 130 incident reports was it one. It was always multiple IEDs. Most civilian tech bomb people may have one or two bombs in their lifetime. But Tom disarmed several hundred in a brief amount of time."

Tim also learned that, even before Tom went, the EOD units from Camp Lejeune had been suffering increasingly high casualty numbers.

"The team that went before Tom's had a 50 percent mortality rate, killed or wounded," Tim said. "So Tom and the people he went over with knew that. That takes a different type of person. If I knew there was a fifty-fifty chance of not coming back with all my belongings and parts, it would take a little more courage to actually go on another tour."

Carolee never shared her concerns with Tom. He had more than enough on his mind in Afghanistan. In addition, this was his first postdivorce deployment, so he had his daughter to worry about as well. Hoping to be supportive, Carolee and Tim planned to be in North Carolina when Tom's unit returned in May 2012.

But on January 16, not long after waking up, Carolee noticed a message on their landline answering machine. She went about her business, only listening to the message later. "Casualty had asked if I could contact them, and I remember yelling for Tim, he was across the way in the other room, because I could not write the number down, the phone number to casualty. I kept playing it over and over again, and I couldn't write it down. I couldn't do it." When the family did call back, she was so upset she couldn't talk to the Marine who answered. "I knew, emotionally, it was bad, but I didn't know what it was and I had to ask them, 'Can you talk to my husband, because I am not going to remember what you're going to tell me?' "

Tim recalls that initial rundown of injuries: two legs had been amputated, one above the knee and one below; they weren't sure they could save his left arm; Tom had suffered a severe penetrating brain injury; and a part of his skull had been removed to allow the brain to swell.

The next call came a little later, from Brian Murphy, a Marine friend of Tom's then stationed in North Carolina. The two had met in Iraq, after the Humvee Murphy had been riding in was blown up. Tom jumped down with his machine gun to provide cover from attacking insurgents until a medevac helicopter arrived. Once Murphy heard about Tom's injuries, he contacted the Ryans, offering to help in any way he could. "Murphy believed that Tom pulled his ass out of the fire, and he wanted to give back," Tim said.

The family was having trouble deciding how to proceed. Tom was being sent to Landstuhl in Germany, and would eventually fly to the States, either landing in California or Washington. But the family didn't know when he would arrive. Plus, in January, flights out of Alaska are canceled frequently because of the weather. It wouldn't be easy to just hop on a plane when word came about Tom's destination. The family was certain about one thing: they weren't going to Landstuhl. "I did not want to go to Germany," Carolee said, with Tim adding, "We always felt that if you're going to Germany, it doesn't look good."

Murphy provided some relief, promising to meet Tom when he arrived at Walter Reed. In the meantime, the Ryans made their way to Seattle, where they would have better access to more flights. And Carolee was calling Germany nonstop. "One night, it was like midnight, but eight o'clock in the morning there, and I just asked the nurse if they could give Tom the phone, and she's like, 'Ma'am, he's not moving.' I'm like, 'Give him the phone. This is his mom. I want to talk to him.' She put it to his ear and I was talking to Tom, knowing that he couldn't talk. I knew that he was in a coma, but that was the first time she had seen movement out of him. He started to move around because he could hear my voice."

Murphy was true to his word. He was at Walter Reed when Tom arrived, and he stayed with his wounded friend in the ICU. He also met the Ryans at the airport when they finally made it to Washington—five days after the blast. He helped them navigate both hospital and city their first few days in the capital. "We were the only parents with our own personal uniformed Marine escort," Tim joked. "In fact, when Murphy left to go home, we didn't know where to go because all we'd had to do was follow him everywhere we went."

Carolee prepared herself to walk into the ICU. "I was a mess, but I knew I had to be strong when I went into his room, for him," Carole said. "He was definitely a mess. I don't think we were prepared to see the severity of it."

They'd heard about the major injuries, the amputations and the head wound, but there was more. His eyes were patched, and they learned that the right eye and optic nerve were gone, though doctors thought they'd be able to save some of the left eye. He had a fractured jaw, a fractured thumb, and fractured clavicle and scapula. Fortunately, none of his internal organs had been injured.

"I was not prepared," Carolee said. "I think that we all live in a world that we think, 'Oh, yeah, they're going to get injured and, yeah, things are going to happen,' but I don't think the real world and us as a family realized the damage that could be done to somebody's body."

They marveled at the military's ability to keep someone with such severe wounds alive, from the battlefield to the aid station to the hospital. "The level of care now is remarkable," Tim said. "My dad was a Navy corpsman in the Korean War, and they couldn't save people like they can now." Carolee added: "When they go out in the field, these guys are prepared for this type of injury. They know what they're supposed to do if somebody's got amputations. They're prepared for it in EOD."

The family was with Tom sometimes from 5:30 a.m. until very late in the night. They were there through shift changes, when Tom was wheeled off to surgery to have his wounds cleaned, and as the staff addressed what seemed like "minor" issues, such as the jaw fracture.

"There were days that were very frantic and stressful, because they didn't know the unknown," Carolee said. Tim adds, "They told us that physically he was fine, because he didn't have any internal injuries. But they were also trying to tell us not to expect too much on the brain recovery. They were basically trying to tell us that he may or may not improve at all."

Communicating with Tom was impossible at first, in part because he was so heavily sedated. In the brief interludes when he did come to, his struggles and anxiety added to his parents' stress.

"The poor guy came to and he had one arm and one hand, and he was completely blind and couldn't hear very well," Tim said. "He would track different voices; you could see him in his bed looking around. He couldn't talk. He was totally overstimulated; he was somewhat terrified of the treatment he was getting. He didn't know where he was, he didn't know how he got there, and nothing seemed to work except for one arm."

Carolee added, "Part of it was that they bring people in, and it wouldn't be one team, it would be many teams for each individual. And they would also have medical students; it's a teaching-learning facility here. And we got it, but we had a young man who, when he was coherent, couldn't see people at all. He was highly sedated, he had no clue what was going on, and people were talking all the time. Nobody was being quiet."

The tension sometimes led to clashes with staff. One nurse made a comment about Carolee's use of hand sanitizer. It was something Carolee did religiously, in addition to being gowned up to enter Tom's room, because of her experience as a certified nursing assistant. "I don't know what she said, but I was in tears," Carolee said. "Tim took me out of the room; she just made me so mad. I just had to leave. I said, 'I don't want her working with my son anymore.' " Looking back, Carolee says, "Part of it was the emotions that I was feeling at the time. I was always washing my hands because I knew, 'infections, infections, infections.' The lady didn't know I knew that. But I'm his mom. I want nothing but the best care." Another time, she showed up in the middle of the night to check on Tom, and there was no nurse in sight. "I had prewarned her before I left that I get these feelings and may come up to the hospital out of the blue if I feel like there's a problem," Carolee said. "And she had left my son, and oh, my God, I was so mad."

The brain injury complicated the recovery process.

Tim said, "For months we had to tell him every day, 'Tom, you're in America now. You're in a hospital. You got blown up by an IED.' We'd only have him for a brief amount of time, and we could ask him, 'Tom, do you know the name of your daughter? Do you know your sisters' names? Do you know this or that?' And then they'd come in and pump some more drugs in him and you'd lose him again. For the longest time you'd have five or ten minutes."

At times, Tom was hallucinating, thinking he was back in Afghanistan. He'd tell his parents he was loading his truck. Or he was upset because he'd marked the IEDs on his hospital room floor and he could hear the nurses walking right over them. He was seeing rabbits and frogs in his room.

It was his Marine friends—Dustin Johns, at Walter Reed recovering from his own injuries, and Brian Murphy—who first helped Tom break the communications barrier. They got him to raise his hand up, moving it one way for "no," and the other for "yes." It was a breakthrough, Carolee recalled. "He was communicating." But, Tim added, "It was brief, right up until the next meds went in."

"They didn't know how much they needed to keep giving him because of all the amputations," Carolee said. "The doctors did not want you in pain, and because Tom couldn't communicate they didn't know how much to give him."

As far back as Germany, when staff tried to lessen his medications to see if he could communicate, Tom became combative. He was put under anesthesia again, to keep him calm and ensure he didn't hurt himself. "I guess getting blown up will put you in a foul mood," Tom would joke later as he heard his parents tell that story.

The family tried to take charge of Tom's environment, turning off lights and playing soothing music. This calmed him, judging by the monitors that measured his heart rate and pulse. They also tried limiting access to the room. "You could see his pulse, for one, would be rapid when there were a lot of people in the room," Tim said. "And when there were fewer people in the room, it would slow down and be calm."

For a time, Tom was pawing at his head, ripping out stitches and trying to remove the patches from his eyes. "I don't think he knew what he was doing," Carolee said. "He just knew something was there." The hospital's initial idea was to tie his remaining hand down, in case they couldn't watch his every move. Absolutely not, Carolee said. "I just thought, 'How would he feel being tied up?' For all he knew he was tied up with insurgents. I don't know what he was thinking at the time." Instead, the family would calmly ask him, over and over, to stop, to please lower his arm. "And he would," Carolee said. "He would bring it back down—very gently."

The family wanted the staff to make more of an effort to communicate with Tom, to find out what he wanted, to determine, as much as possible, the extent of his brain damage. Instead, they thought there was too much emphasis on preparing them for a worst-case scenario. "If that's how Tom was going to be, fine. I would've dealt with that," Carolee said. "But then, nobody really knew what was going on. Why just assume? We didn't know, but I didn't think that was how Tom was going to be. And I know my child better than anybody else does."

They began consulting with the Department of Veterans Affairs, and researching polytrauma hospitals. "We asked for options," Carolee said. Six weeks after the blast, they had Tom moved to the Richmond Polytrauma Rehabilitation Center, one of five facilities around the country that helps vets and service members with multiple traumas, whether physical—such as amputations—or brain injuries. It was exactly what the Ryans were searching for.

"The doctors pulled us in to see what we were looking at," Carolee recalled. "Then they were going to start weaning Tom off his narcotics because they said his brain will never ever heal if he's on narcotics. They wanted to know what we wanted out of this whole thing, and they talked to Tom, to see what he wanted."

With his jaw healing and unwired, speech therapy started almost immediately. Tim described it: "You got sixty seconds to name as many states in America as you can, starting now. Or you have exactly one minute to name as many pieces of fruit. Or, Tom, you've gone to a restaurant and you've eaten your meal and it's time to pay the check. But you find out you've left your wallet at home. What do you do?"

At first, Tom was still in bed for everything. He was too weak to move himself to a chair or a commode. Even when he could get around more,

Tom learned just how weak he'd become when his physical therapy started. "I was pretty much skin and bones," Tom recalled. "The guy handed me a five-pound weight when I first went in there, and I said, 'Five pounds? You handed me a five-pound weight? That's almost insulting.' Come to find out, I'd been in a hospital bed so long it was hard to lift a five-pound weight." By the time he left Richmond, six weeks after his arrival, he could transfer himself in and out of a one-handed wheelchair.

Still blind, though starting to see shapes out of his left eye, Tom started to gain back some independence by relearning to care for himself. He was taught how to line up his toothbrush, toothpaste, razor, and other items on his sink, the same exact way every time, so he knew where things were and could get himself ready for the day.

The road to independence begins with small and simple steps that can make all the difference.

"It's definitely a learning curve," Carolee said. "Tom's been independent and on his own since he was eighteen, and I'm sure he can tell you how it feels that all of a sudden your mother is here to take care of you when you used to be able to take care of yourself and your daughter."

"That doesn't even describe the worst," Tom replies. "The 'not even going to the bathroom by yourself,' literally not being able to go to the bathroom or take a shower by yourself, that was humbling. From doing everything I've ever done and all that, and then coming out of being drugged, and I can't even go to the bathroom by myself. Everyone is worried that I'll fall down."

Of course, being so close after so many years apart can mean learning things one would rather not know. For example, when Carolee saw a picture of a scantily clad Tom on Facebook, taken when his unit was celebrating the end of a deployment, her reaction was: "My son's in a cheetah thong. Lord, help us." Tom laughs at the memory: "The funniest thing was that was the first thing she noticed. First thing I noticed was, 'Wow, I look so young and I have nice legs.' "

When he entered Richmond, Tom's mom was still calling the shots for his care. Six weeks later, he was able to pass a test that meant he could be in charge. "That was our goal," Tim said, "to get him back to the point where he had a little more independence, a little more control."

"It's a really different environment than Walter Reed," Tom said. "It's all on one floor, and the doctors don't rotate out, and all the staff stays the same. And that's all they do—severe head injuries, and with multiple traumas. They're very good about knowing what people need. They were willing to work with me on pain medications, taking me off this stuff that was making me hallucinate. They had to remedicate me but it was stuff that didn't make you hallucinate, didn't make you just zone out in bed."

Some of the pain that returned was different. "I could tell it wasn't normal pain," Tom said, "It was all phantom pain. It's when you have pain in your limbs that are no longer there, and I guess it's caused from your brain trying to send messages down there and there's nothing there, so your body interprets it as pain. But it can be brutal, it really can."

Carolee and Tim saw another important difference at the Polytrauma Center. "In Richmond, everybody that deals with the individual meets on a regular basis," Tim said, with Carolee adding, "Once a week." He continued, "And they all know what's going on with that individual every single day."

Three months after he was wounded, with Tom ready to return to Walter Reed to start learning to use prosthetic legs, Richmond had provided the Ryans with an answer about the extent of his brain injury. And it was far from the worst.

"We learned along the way that Tom is pretty intelligent, extremely intelligent in certain things," his mom said. "But it's just going to take him a little longer to process things, and we've learned that we can't say, 'Tom, you need to do this, this, this, and this.' That just sets him in an overwhelming world and he doesn't know where to start."

One step at a time he can handle though, and that described life back at Walter Reed, as he began using prosthetic legs. Even this would be complicated, first with an infection that made walking with prosthetics excruciatingly painful for months, and also by constant dizziness while walking, likely a result of his vision problems and brain injury.

"For somebody who is amputated above the knee on both legs, they start you out on shorties," Tom explained. "Shorties are as short as you can make them. It'll be your socket plus three to four inches of pylon. They make them as short as they can so you can get your balance back, and get used to being upright—and learn how to get yourself back up when you fall down. The shorter you are, the easier it is to get back up."

And he stresses this last point with a smile: "You fall down all the time. We're professionals at falling down."

If the service member is missing two legs, he can start with shorties and two canes for balance. In Tom's case, he was given a prosthetic left arm with a cane attached. "I finally gave that up because it hurt my back," he said. "It was making me bend over, so I just went to one cane."

Gradually, the legs become longer. "He's taller than me now," Carolee notes. "Yeah," Tom agrees, "but that's since I got my knees. It took me from April to, I guess in December or January I got my knees, so that's a long time I was on shorties. And they don't have knees. They don't bend. You're just walking around stiff-legged."

Tom works on walking five days a week, about an hour a day. "Some people spend all day down there," Tom noted. "I don't usually do more than an hour a day. It's exhausting, and I have problems with my sockets."

Sockets are the shell that encases a liner-covered limb and connects the user to the prosthesis.

Fitting a normal socket for Tom's right stump, which is higher than on his left and a different shape, proved problematic. There are belts to secure them, but they are difficult for a one-armed person to maneuver. As Tom said, if the sockets don't fit properly, "it's like standing in five-gallon buckets."

"Initially I started with a normal socket, and then I had to change that because it was just falling off," Tom said. "It's a problem that people with shorter limbs tend to have. I really didn't have enough leg to keep it on, so it was just falling off. And then they went to a pin lock, where the liner that you wear has a pin on it and that locks into the bottom of the socket. That stayed on better but it would start ripping my liner off when I fell down. It would just tear off my leg. And then I went on a walking strike. I said, 'Hey, we have to find a solution to this because it just rips the liner off and there's no point in me walking in circles and being frustrated.' So I quit walking, and they got me a different socket, which works a lot better."

Microprocessor-controlled knee joints, which cost about $30,000 apiece—"I'm walking on a whole bunch of expensive stuff," Tom said—take him from the stiff-legged gait of shorties to even being able to walk up stairs. "It's programmed to where you make a certain jerking movement, and it turns off the hydraulics, so you step up onto a stair," Tom said. "In other words, you 'break' the knee and then it turns off the hydraulics so you can step up. And then going down, you take and put the heel of whichever leg you're going to lower yourself on, the last couple inches of your heel on the edge of the step, and then you put all your weight on it, and it just slowly lowers you down."

They can be adapted to the user, but the "you fall down all the time" rule still applies: "They're programmable," Tom said. "They can change how much weight you have to put onto it for it to go down, how fast it lowers you, or how slow it lowers you. But my left one didn't work the last time, and I got a face full of ground."

Uneven ground, even a slightly slanting sidewalk, also presents problems. "They can be a little temperamental on uneven ground," Tom said. "Trying to walk across a slanted area is where I actually have a hard time. It's weird, because I'm walking fine in one direction, but if I turn around and come back, I'm probably going to fall down. I think it has to do with the fact that I'm way more confident using my left leg than my right one because I have more control over my leg with the longer stump."

His new home in North Carolina will include paths from his house to the barn that will make caring for his horses easier. And he'll also have a track chair, which comes with treads that allow users to get out in the woods for hunting—Tom's came with a gun rack. The challenge is how best to adapt to a new reality, with maximum independence, both for Tom and Aidan, while recognizing certain limitations.

Carolee has certainly done her share of adapting. A month after Tom returned to Walter Reed from Richmond, she went back to Juneau for her daughter's wedding. Becca had considered canceling because Tom couldn't be there, but her mom talked her out of it. It's not what her brother would want, even if he couldn't make the trip. While at home, Carolee visited her workplace, SERCC, which provides support services to students, school districts, and communities. The staff had been very supportive of her and her family since Tom's injury, and assumed that Carolee would return when she was ready. They were surprised to learn that the purpose of her visit was to turn her keys in. "They didn't realize the intensity of the whole thing," Carolee said. "I knew in my heart I couldn't go back to work and leave my son here."

There would be no return to life as it was.

"It was the hardest day, to give up my job," Carolee said, brushing back a tear. "I knew that I needed to do it, but just knowing that I was moving on to something else in my life, that I was not moving back to Juneau … That's not a bad thing. It's just that we're changing and going in a different route now. Tom needs me. Aidan needs me."

That different route has had some surprising twists and turns, especially when it comes to Tom's progress. A year after Becca's wedding, it was his sister Jessica's turn. She and her fiancé had also planned a wedding in Juneau, but now things were different. Tom had made dramatic improvements. Sight had gradually been returning to his left eye and, despite some problems, he was considerably more adept at walking on prosthetics. The couple decided to move the wedding to Tom.

"He walked his little sister down the aisle, with my husband," Carolee said. "It was very sweet."

It was also a validation of Carolee's time at Walter Reed, and her belief that her family played a crucial role in Tom's recovery. "It's extremely important to have family around for them to succeed," Carolee said. "Yes, they are going to have challenges, and yes, everybody is going to be frustrated. But we'll get through it. I mean, he could've died, easily. But I have my son here. So whatever we have to get through, we can get through it. It may not be pretty one day, but we will get through it."

SIX

ROBERT SCOTT III AND VALENCE SCOTT

R OBERT SCOTT III MISSED THE 7:37 A.M. LONG ISLAND RAIL ROAD TRAIN on that sunny morning while heading to work in New York City on September 11, 2001. The elegantly handsome young man was preparing for his usual workday as a trader specialist clerk for Goldman Sachs, one of the most well-respected investment houses on Wall Street. Thankfully, for his mother, Valence, his tardiness was a blessing. Robert lost fifteen of his friends following the terrorist attacks that leveled both of the World Trade Center towers, left the Pentagon in flames, and saw Flight 93 crash in Shanksville, Pennsylvania. This was the worst act of terror on US soil since the bombing of Pearl Harbor on December 7, 1941.

The nation was in shock. This unimaginable tragedy mobilized many young men and women who wanted to serve their country and go after the terrorists who had inflicted so much pain on the United States. Not since World War II was there such an outpouring of patriotism, pride, defiance, and outrage that such inhumane acts could be inflicted.

Robert and his family were devastated by the attack in the city they love, and suffered the pain of losing so many of their close friends. Over the next year Robert kept thinking about the way he could get involved, and his solution was to join the military. He enlisted in the US Army, hoping to avenge the deaths of his friends and prevent the bad guys from inflicting even more terror on American soil.

Robert had a tremendous capacity for retaining information and logically thinking through almost any situation. His mind was his machine.

That's why he was such an accomplished trader, and why he was assigned to intelligence work after basic training.

Today, when asked, he can't remember what clothes he wore the day before, if he ate his dinner, or even if he took a shower.

Robert Scott III had been a serious student, earning two degrees from Norfolk State University in finance and economics. His dream was to be an accountant, but after he did an internship on the trading floor of Goldman Sachs, he fell in love with the trading profession and decided to make it his vocation. Robert looked the part, too. Always impeccably dressed, he took pride in his appearance, and when he walked confidently into a room, people noticed. "Robert always liked to match up his clothes. He was always neat and put together," Valence said.

Daphne, too, couldn't help but notice this young man's charisma. She was his girlfriend, a woman who eventually became his wife and the mother of his son, Robert IV.

Robert had excelled at Goldman Sachs, which meant a lot to the tight-knit Scott family. Family means everything to Valence and her husband, Robert Jr.

"It was love at first sight," Valence said of her husband. "When I met my husband forty-one years ago, we had an immediate connection. I made sure that on our first date I was dressed to the nines. I had hair down to my waist and was wearing a gorgeous dress; I could see he was hooked." And why wouldn't he be? This petite spitfire, with a hybrid Jamaican/Long Island accent, could charm anyone with her beaming smile and alluring figure.

Robert was the couple's only child, and they lived in Long Island, New York. Though Valence was originally born in Jamaica, she and her family came to the US to build a better life, and for Valence to further her education. She studied at the Washington Business Institute in New York, earning a degree in business and human resources. After college, she started a new adventure of her own—working as a human resources and benefits professional. Life for the Scotts was good. The American dream was their reality.

Then came September 11, and the decision that would dramatically change all of their lives forever.

Robert said that the previous evening's football game was the reason he missed the train that morning.

"My dad and I were watching a football game and we stayed up late," Robert said. "My mom was sick and stayed home from work that day, so I

Chapter 1: Mark Fidler and Stacy Fidler

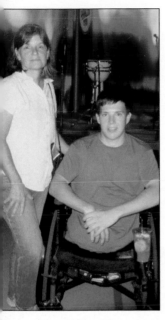

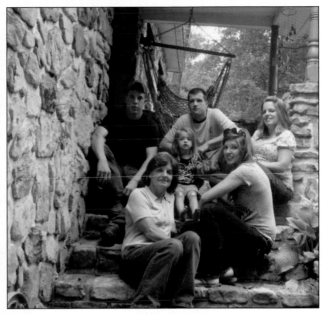

Mark and Stacy Fidler at Tim
McGraw's concert in Washington, DC.

Mark and his family enjoy a day together at home in Pennsylvania.
Top row: Mark, Mark's brother-in-law (Bill), and Mark's sister (Amanda).
Bottom row: Stacy, her granddaughter (Alyssa), and Mark's other sister (Kelly).

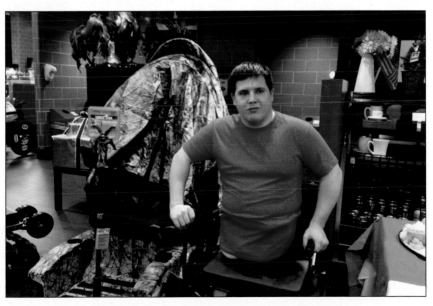

Mark goes shopping on Black Friday at the Navy Exchange.

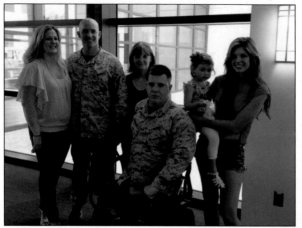

The Fidler family celebrates Mark's promotion to Corporal. Joining him for this honor were: Brittany Dittmer-Fidler, Dan Fidler, Stacy Fidler, and Kelly Fidler.

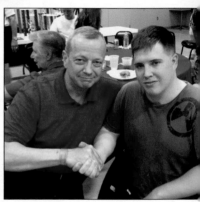

Mark and Marine General John Allen (Ret.) at an event held for Mark by Faces of Valor, which does a major fund-raiser every year to support a wounded warrior. General Allen and his family showed up to support Mark. Credit: Dava Gueri

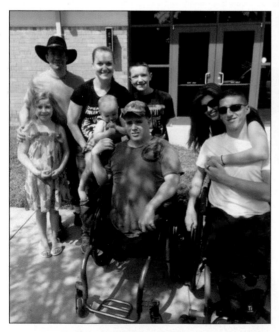

Supporting Mark at his Faces of Valor fund-raiser in Annapolis, Maryland, left to right: Steven Brewer, Lorelei Brewer, Chelle McIntyre-Brewer, Killian Brewer, Cavan Brewer, Mark Fidler, Kelly Fidler, and Timothy William Donley. Credit: Dava Guerin.

Chapter 2: Josh Brubaker and Mary Brubaker

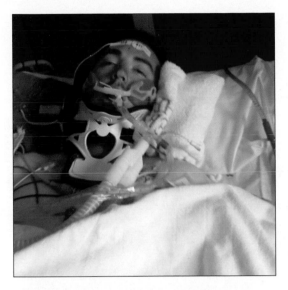

Josh Brubaker in the hospital at Walter Reed.

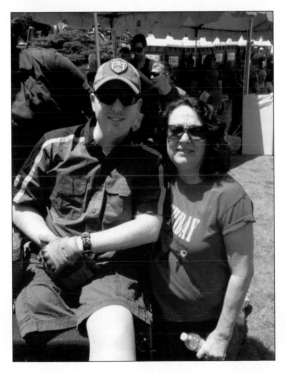

Josh and Mary Brubaker attend Gary Sinise's Invincible Spirit Festival at Walter Reed.

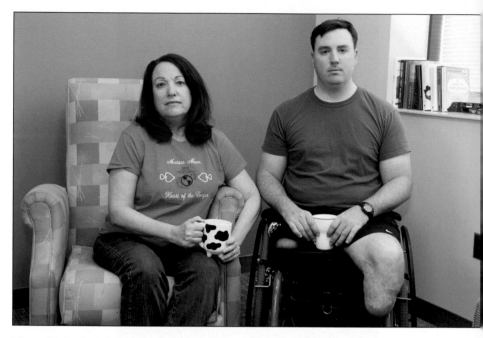

Mary and Josh relax before getting ready for the day ahead. Credit: Josh Ghering.

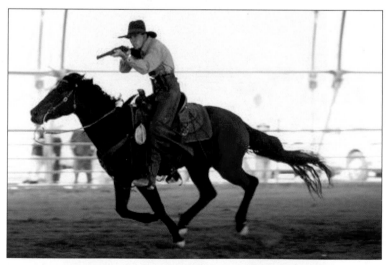

Josh competes in a Cowboy Mounted Shooting Association event.

Chapter 3: Christian Brown and Lyn Braden-Reed

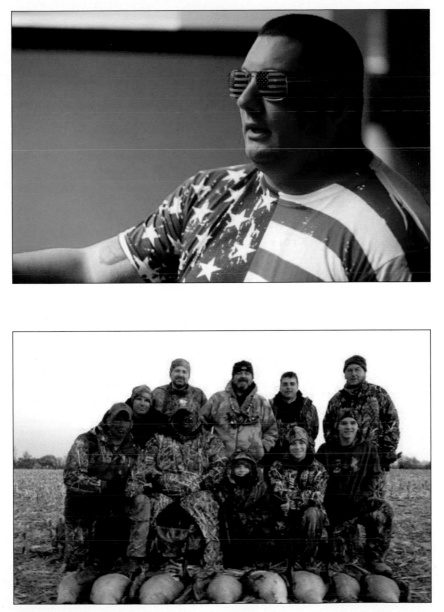

Christian and his hunting buddies.

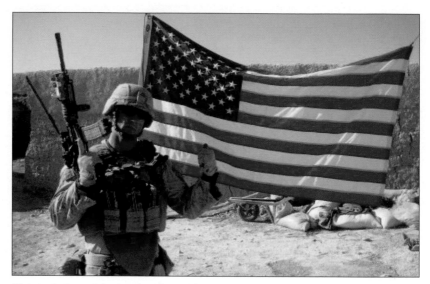

Christian in front of the American flag in Afghanistan.

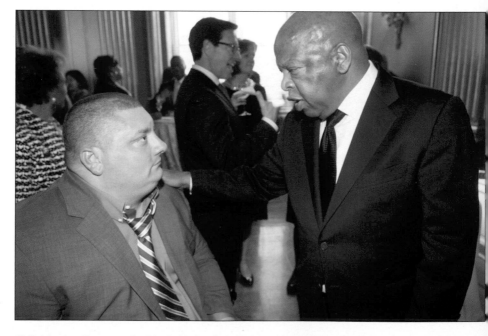

Civil rights icon Representative John Lewis spends some time with Christian at the US Association of Former Members of Congress's Statesmanship Awards Dinner. Credit: Josh Ghering.

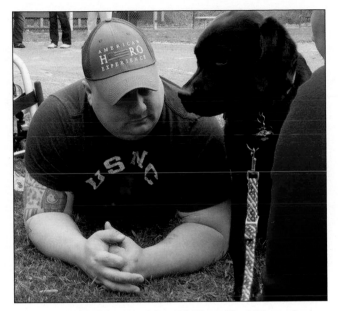

Christian Brown shares a light moment with "Puppy Derek," the service dog named after Siobhan Fuller-McConnell's son Derek McConnell.

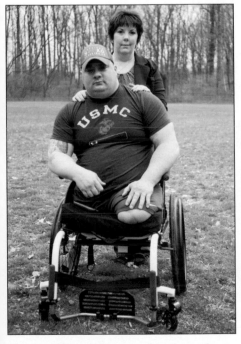

Christian and his mom, Lyn, enjoy the spring weather at a baseball field in Bethesda, Maryland. Credit: Josh Ghering.

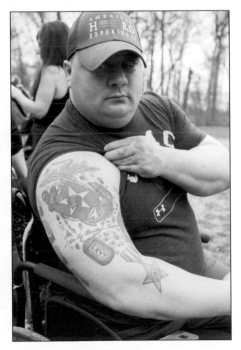

Christian proudly shows off his tattoos. Credit: Josh Ghering.

Chapter 4: Tyler Jeffries and Pam Carrigan Britt

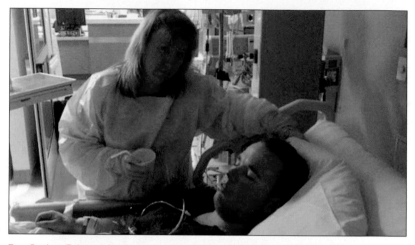

Pam Carrigan Britt standing by her son Tyler Jeffries at Walter Reed.

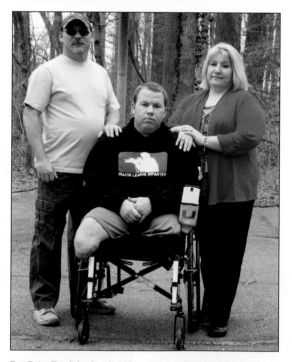

Ray Britt (Pam's husband), Tyler, and Pam. Credit: Josh Ghering.

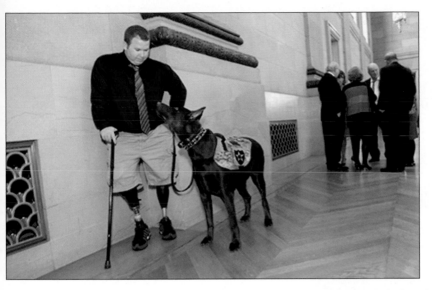

Tyler and his service dog, Apollo, take a break at the Mellon Auditorium in Washington, DC. Credit: Josh Ghering.

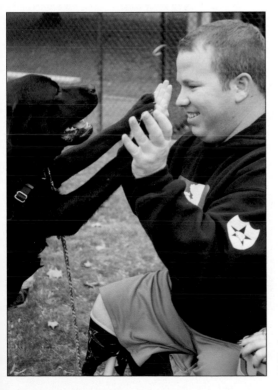

Tyler and the service dog named after
Derek McConnell at a baseball field in Bethesda,
Maryland. Credit: Josh Ghering.

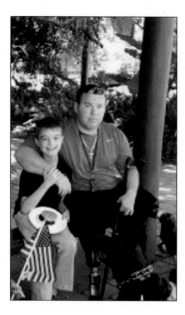

Tyler visits an elementary school in Florida to surprise eight-year-old student Lucas Giese, who has been sending letters and care packages to Tyler at Walter Reed almost every week for two years. He and Tyler are great friends, and the relationship has helped both of them.

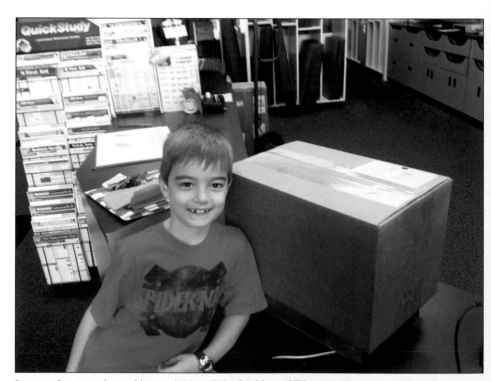

Lucas sends a care package to his pen pal Tyler at Walter Reed from a UPS store in Florida. November 2012.

Chapter 5: Thomas McRae and Carolee Ryan

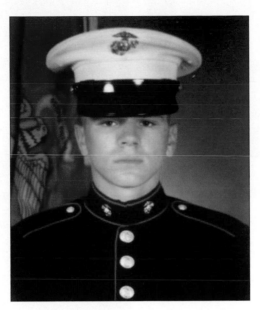

Staff Sergeant Thomas McRae.

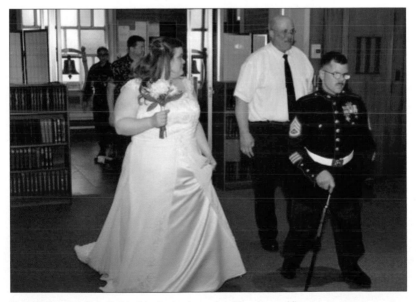

Tom McRae proudly walks his sister Jessica down the aisle at her wedding.

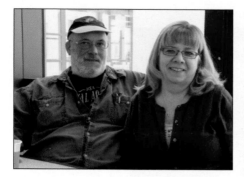

Tom's parents Carolee Ryan and Tim Ryan at the Warrior Café.

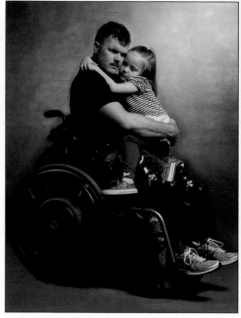

Tom and his daughter, Aidan.

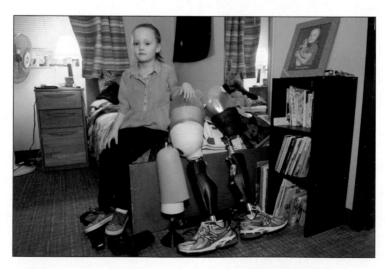

Tom's daughter, Aidan, poses with his prosthetic legs. Credit: Josh Ghering.

Chapter 6: Robert Scott III and Valence Scott

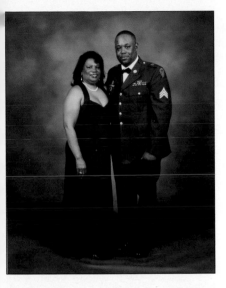

Valence Scott and her son, Robert Scott III, enjoy a night out on the town.

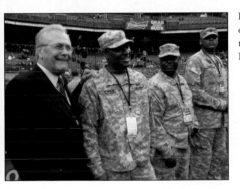

Robert and his fellow wounded soldiers are guests of honor at Yankee Stadium for the 9/11 Memorial tribute along with former Secretary of Defense Donald Rumsfeld.

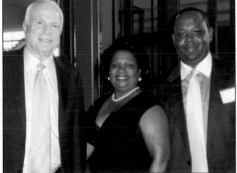

Robert and Valence attend a wounded warrior brunch in Washington, DC, with Senator John McCain.

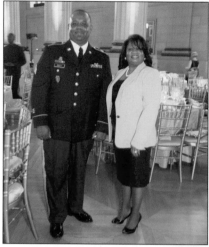

Robert and Valence dressed to the nines for a much-needed night out. They and all of the Mighty Moms and their wounded warriors were guests at a dinner in Washington, DC. Credit: Josh Ghering.

Robert is the guest of the New York Giants football team.

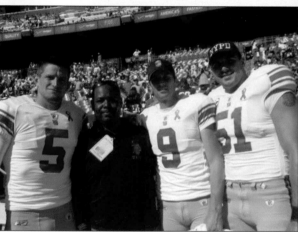

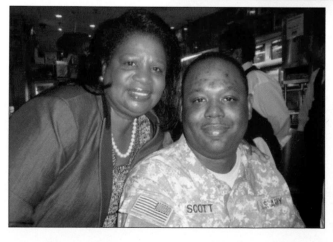

Valence enjoys an evening out with Robert at a wounded warrior dinner.

Chapter 7: Jeffrey Shonk and Tammy Karcher

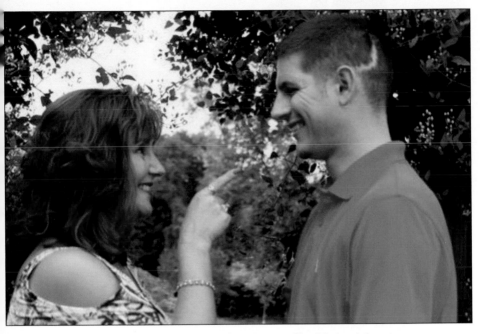

Tammy Karcher and her son, Jeffrey Shonk, share a light moment outside of the hospital.

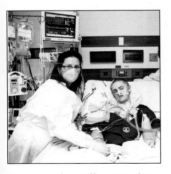

Tammy comforts Jeffrey soon after his arrival at Walter Reed.

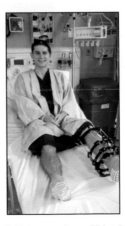

Jeffrey recovering at Walter Reed National Military Medical Center.

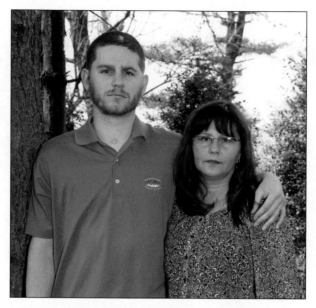

Jeffrey and Tammy together, as they have been for many years. Credit: Josh Ghering.

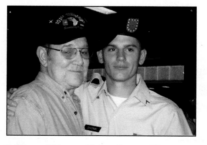

Jeffrey and his grandfather George Glenn.

Chapter 8: Adam Keys and Julie Keys

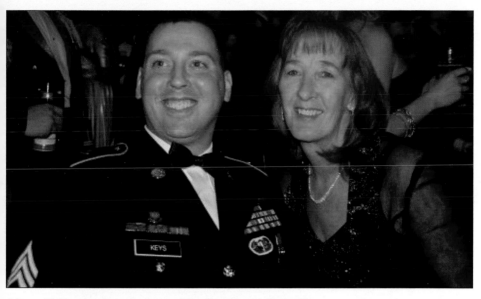

Adam and Julie getting the royal treatment at President Obama's inauguration.

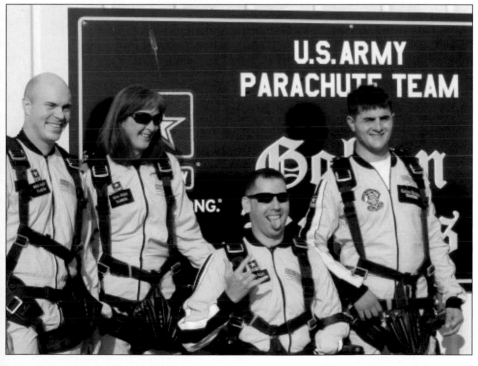

Julie and Adam doing a parachute jump with the US Army Parachute Team.

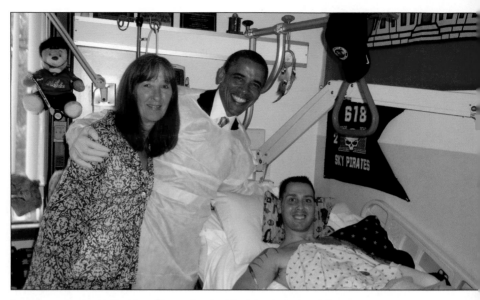

Julie shares a laugh with President Obama when he visits Adam in the hospital.

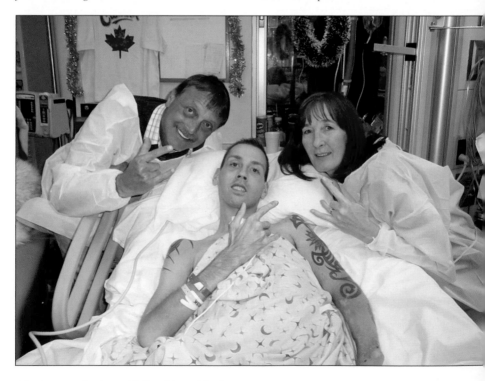

Adam's parents, Stephen and Julie, celebrate Adam's return.

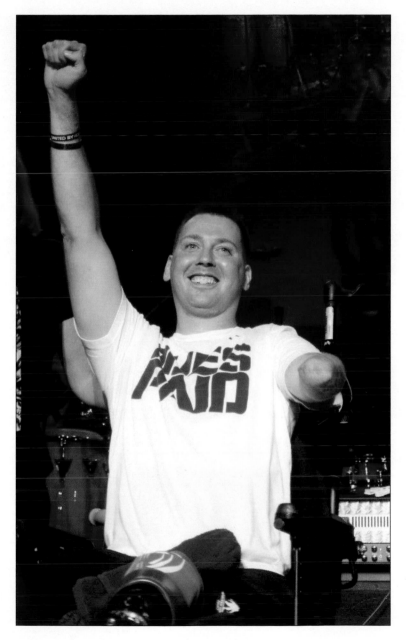
Adam thanks his guests at a benefit concert given in his honor.

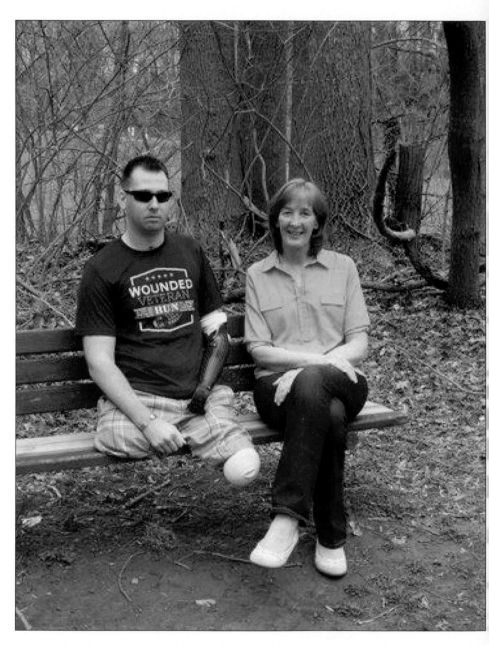

Julie and Adam relaxing on a park bench in Bethesda, Maryland.

Chapter 9: Stefanie D. Mason and Paulette Mason

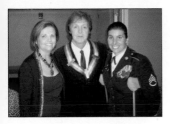

Paulette and Stefanie Mason meet Beatle Paul McCartney in the Presidential Reception Suite at the Kennedy Center Honors event.

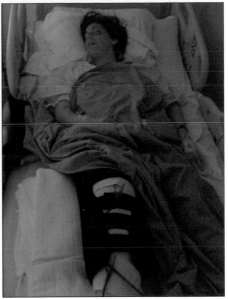

Stefanie after she arrived from Afghanistan to Walter Reed.

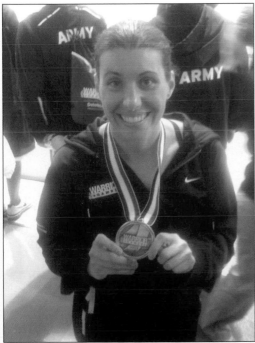

A gold medal for Staff Sergeant Stefanie Mason at the Wounded Warrior Games, Olympic Village, in Colorado.

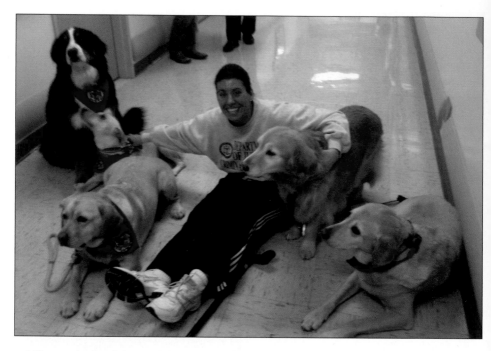

Military service dogs help wounded warriors through their therapy. Here Stefanie plays with them in the hall at Walter Reed.

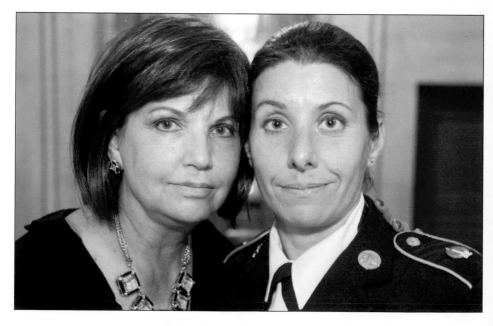

Paulette Mason and her daughter Stefanie.

Chapter 10: Derek McConnell and Siobhan Mary Fuller-McConnell, Esq.

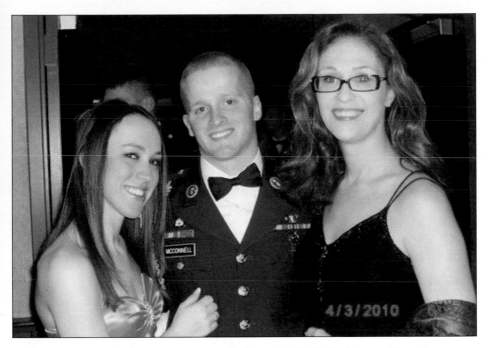

Siobhan Fuller-McConnell and her son Derek McConnell's fiancée, Krystina, join Derek for a special event in Washington, DC.

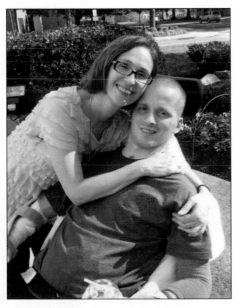

Siobhan and Derek share a tender moment during a trip outside of Walter Reed.

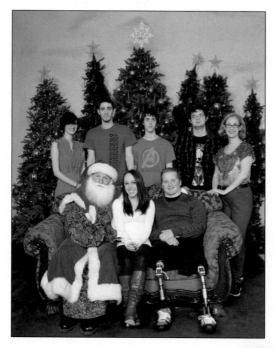

Siobhan, Derek, Krystina, and the family at Christmas.

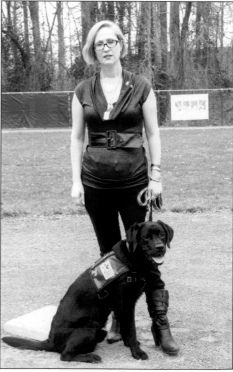

Siobhan spends some quality time with the service dog
"Puppy Derek," named after her son Derek.
Credit: Josh Ghering.

Chapter 11: Band of Mothers

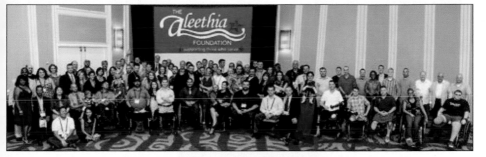

Mighty Moms and their wounded warriors take part in the Aleethia Foundation's popular Friday night dinners.

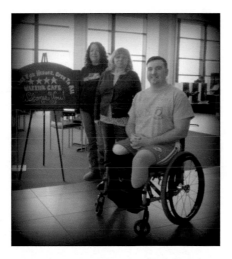

Mary Brubaker, Carolee Ryan, and Josh Brubaker
at the Warrior Café.

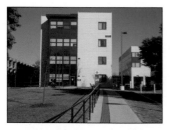

Outside of Building 62 at Walter Reed.

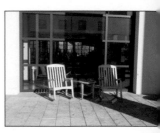

Moms' rocking chairs in front of Building 62.

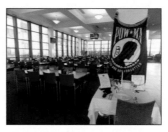

The Warrior Café.

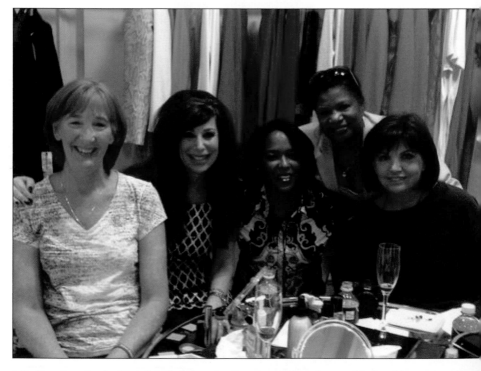

Julie Keys, Dava Guerin, Felecia Suluki of Operation Homefront, Valence Scott, and Paulette Mason enjoy a day of beauty at Saks Fifth Avenue in Chevy Chase, Maryland.

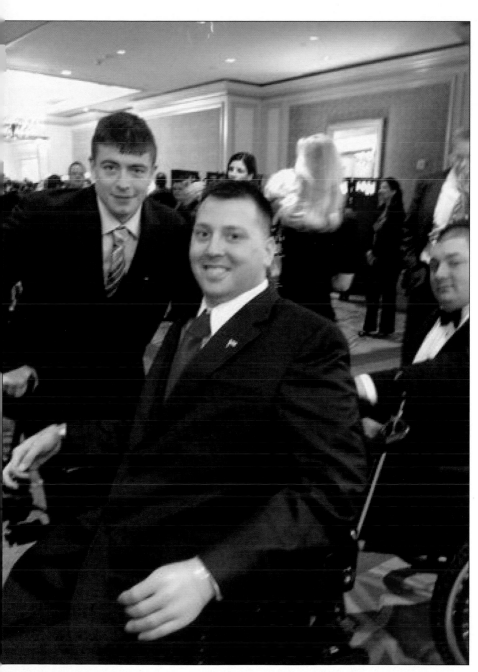

Mark Wasylenko, Adam Keys, and Christian Brown hanging out.

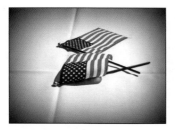

Flags at the Gary Sinise Foundation's
Invincible Spirit Festival at Walter Reed.

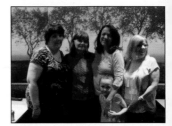

Lyn, Stacy, Mary, Carolee, and Aidan
take part in the "See Ya Later" party in
honor of Mary and Josh leaving Walter
Reed. The moms won't say "good-bye"
since their friendships will be forever.
Credit: Jennifer Magerer.

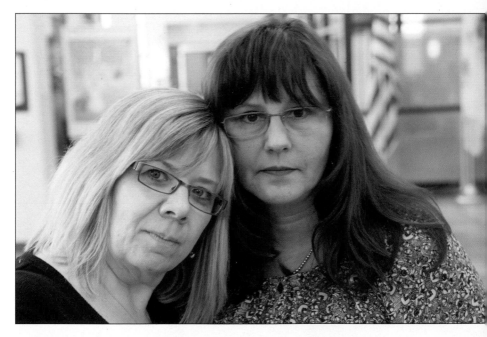

Carolee Ryan and Tammy Karcher have become friends and comfort each other in times of need. Here they share
an intimate moment together. Credit: Josh Ghering.

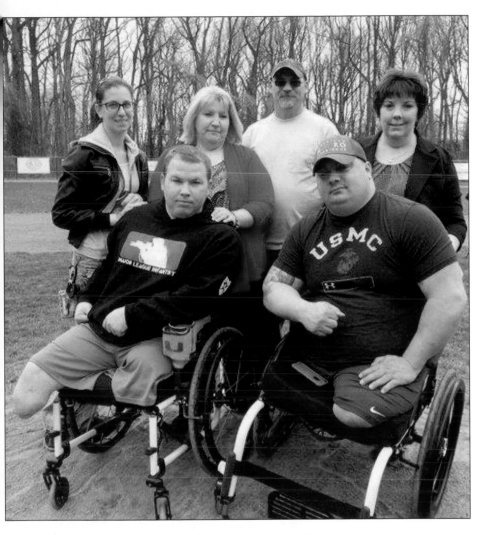

Pam Carrigan Britt, her husband Raymond, Tyler's friend Deidra, and Tyler Jeffries with Lyn Braden-Reed and Christian Brown at a park in Bethesda, Maryland. (Top, from left: Deidra, Pam, Raymond, Lyn; bottom: Tyler and Christian)

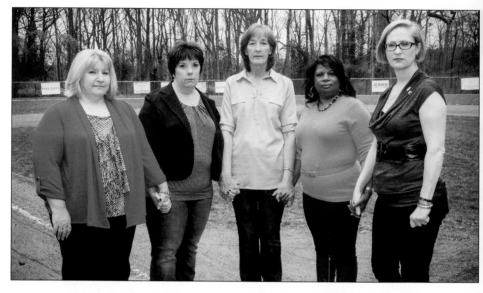

Moms Pam Carrigan Britt, Lyn Braden-Reed, Julie Keys, Valence Scott, and Siobhan Fuller-McConnell. Credit: Josh Ghering.

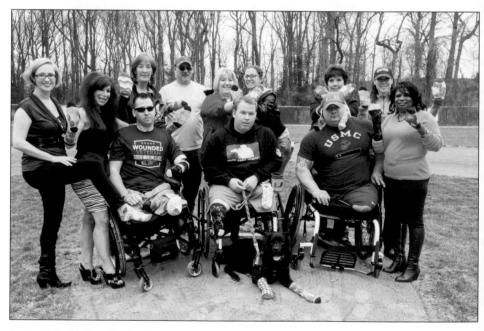

Siobhan Fuller-McConnell, author Dava Guerin, Julie Keys and her son Adam, Ray Britt (Pam Carrigan Britt's husband), Pam, her son Tyler Jeffries, Tyler's friend Deidra Arthur, Lyn Braden-Reed and her son Christian, Jennifer Brusstar (CEO of the Tug McGraw Foundation), and Valence Scott hold up the socks that were used in a photo that was sent to President George H. W. Bush for his ninetieth birthday—although many of the wounded warriors no longer need socks, they still maintain a sense of humor. Credit: Josh Ghering.

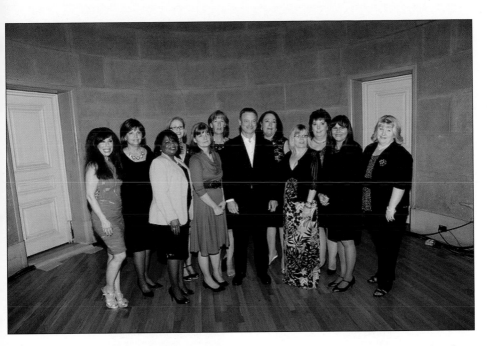

Actor and philanthropist Gary Sinise with all of the Mighty Moms of Walter Reed and author Dava Guerin at the US Association of Former Members of Congress Dinner. From left: Author Dava Guerin, Paulette Mason, Valence Scott, Siobhan Fuller-McConnell, Stacy Fidler, Julie Keys, Mary Brubaker, Carolee Ryan, Lyn Braden-Reed, Tammy Karcher, and Pam Carrigan Britt. Credit: Keith Jewell.

About the Contributors

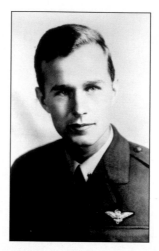

George H. W. Bush, World War II Navy Pilot, August 1942–September 1945. Credit: George Bush Presidential Library and Museum.

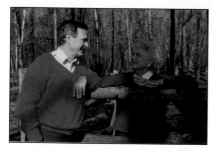

President and Mrs. Bush.

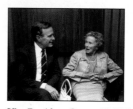

Vice President George H. W. Bush visits his mother, Mrs. Dorothy Walker Bush, while campaigning in Miami, Florida. Credit: George Bush Presidential Library and Museum.

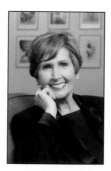

Ambassador Connie Morella.

overslept; that's why I missed the train. I would have been in Tower One when the first plane hit."

"Normally, I am the first one up in the morning, and ironically, on September 11 I was really sick," Valence said. "I had the flu and took some medication so I didn't get out of bed that morning. Had I been better, I would have woken Robert up, and who knows what would have happened. I can't even think about it."

Though saved that day, he could have never imagined that, only eight years later, he would become another tragic statistic of the War on Terror.

After losing fifteen of his friends that day, Robert was devastated and tried to figure out a way he could help in the war effort and avenge the senseless deaths of so many innocent victims. Valence said that Robert came home from work one day and told his parents that he decided to join the Army. "I didn't want Robert to go into the military. He is our only child, and the thought of losing him was devastating," said Valence. But Robert was an adult, and Valence and her husband had to respect his decision.

Nevertheless, the pull to find a meaningful way to support the country was too overwhelming for Robert to ignore. He was more than happy to put the pen to paper. "We were very proud of him, of course, and especially because of what he said to us when he made the decision. He said: 'Ma, it's not about the money; it is about serving my country with honor and pride.'" Valence said those words kept her going throughout her son's deployment, and they would be the source of great comfort after the tragedy that was to come only five years later.

Both Robert's father and grandfather were in the Army, so he was familiar with what it meant to serve. "I knew I would miss Wall Street, but money comes and goes and doesn't need to be spent. I thought that I should just do it, because that's the heart of being an American. Plus, I was a 'Bond kid' and grew up wanting to do intelligence."

Robert put as much dedication and energy into his military career as he did when he worked on Wall Street. He served with pride and loved being an Army intelligence analyst. He completed basic training at Fort Leonard Wood and continued his advanced training in Arizona and Hawaii before deploying to Iraq in 2007. What he actually did in Iraq is still a mystery for Valence and her husband, and that comes as no surprise since he dealt with a "good bit of classified information," Valence recalled.

Ever the devoted and loving son, Robert tried to call his mother as often as he could, and those phone calls gave Valence great comfort and peace. "Our family was always close," Valence said. "We talked about any and all issues, and we have a special bond. I would always say to Robert that 'you're here for me and I'm here for you.'" Those bonds, as well as the bonds Valence developed much later with other moms of wounded warriors, would come to be her salvation.

Robert had only ten days before he was scheduled to come home from Iraq, and Valence and her husband were thrilled that they would see him again.

Before arriving in New York, he would return to his base in Hawaii, where his parents planned to welcome their young hero. Valence was on pins and needles and couldn't contain her excitement, often waking up in the middle of the night as she imagined holding him in her arms and seeing his wide and gentle smile.

Valence had made that trip to Hawaii once before, to take Robert's Army buddies out for lunch at Chili's and thank them for their service. "We had a great time with all of the guys, and we wanted them to know how much we appreciated their service. We wanted to let them know in person that we thought of them as our own sons, too. After lunch, Robert and I went for a drive and bought thirty-six balloons—one for each of his teammates—and then we released them by Oahu Beach to symbolize their courage."

Valence was so excited just thinking about seeing Robert again. They had been able to talk almost every day during his deployment—so she felt his presence even though he was a world away from home. "He was going to be home in February 2009, the twenty-seventh to be exact. I spoke to him that day and he said: 'Ma, we are leaving soon, and I'll call you when I get to the airport.' I said, 'Okay,' and I left my office."

She stopped by the bank to get some cash before getting on her flight to Hawaii. Then the unimaginable happened. "The phone rang, and the person on the other end of the line told me that Robert was in a coma. They asked me the last four digits of my social security number, and I thought it might be a mistake. I asked if they had the right Scott, because that couldn't be Robert since I just talked to him. When I finally told them the number, I knew it was Robert and that something really terrible happened to him."

What happened was this: Robert was traveling in a tank, and suffered a deep vein thrombosis (DVT). Because of the lack of blood flow to his heart and brain, Robert passed out within seconds and was totally unresponsive. According to the Mayo Clinic, a DVT is a condition in which a blood clot forms in one or more of the deep veins in the body. A DVT can cause leg pain, but often occurs without any symptoms. If the blood clot breaks loose it can travel through the bloodstream and lodge in the lungs, blocking blood flow and causing a pulmonary embolism. Sitting for long periods of time in small, cramped spaces, like a military tank or an airplane, can trigger this condition. A DVT caused the death of NBC's Iraq war correspondent David Bloom. Tennis star Serena Williams and singer Lady Gaga also suffered from DVTs, though they survived.

Robert's brain was robbed of oxygen for at least thirty minutes, resulting in a severe brain injury; thankfully, he was still alive.

Like the visible wounds of the wars in Iraq and Afghanistan—such as those suffered from IEDs and other blasts, vehicle accidents, and burns—the unseen injuries, including traumatic brain injuries (TBIs) and post-traumatic stress disorder (PTSD), can be especially devastating. A TBI, usually the result of an external force causing brain dysfunction, can cause dramatic personality changes, affecting a person's ability to speak and control his or her emotions. Other symptoms include depression, insomnia, memory loss, difficulty doing the most basic tasks, and impaired reasoning and judgment, as well as physical conditions such as infection and damage to blood vessels. Every person recovers differently from a TBI, and there is no one-size-fits-all prognosis or treatment.

For Robert, there was just no way to tell how severe his brain damage was.

"I was totally destroyed; I had just spoken to him," Valence said in disbelief. They told Valence that Robert collapsed and they had a hard time reviving him and couldn't get a pulse. Finally, once he was stabilized, he was flown to Germany, where he was treated by military medical professionals who were very familiar with such injuries. "I was calling Germany every ten minutes, trying to find out as much as I could about my son's condition. What was really killing me was imagining my son a half a world away and all alone," Valence said as her voice cracked from the painful memory. "He had nobody with him but God," Valence added.

Valence is a woman of deep faith, and she called upon that faith to help her cope with her worst nightmare. Her only son, her baby, was alone in a foreign land, and she was helpless. For the first time in her life, this bright, take-charge woman was at the mercy of strangers. Her son, Robert, afraid and by himself, was now a statistic of the War on Terror. She was numb.

Valence and her husband were ready to buy their plane tickets to Germany when she received a call informing her that Robert would be flown to Walter Reed. "I will always remember that wonderful woman Theresa—I have to find her someday just to thank her—because she was so kind and caring. She called me and told me to keep calm, and that Robert was in good hands. She said that she would make sure he was not alone and said she knew that too, because she saw God in his eyes." Valence was relieved.

When Valence arrived in Washington, she went right to Walter Reed, and happened to notice an ambulance as she was entering the hospital. "I had a weird feeling that Robert was inside; I was so devastated." She rushed to the ICU but was told she couldn't see Robert for a few hours. "They told us that they had to do a complete workup on him and make sure that he was stable and didn't have any infectious diseases," Valence said. At that point she didn't care what shape Robert was in. She only cared that her son was alive. "At least he was on this side of the world, and I could see him. Just to see his face, and tell him I loved him, was the most wonderful thing for me."

As the extended Scott family began to arrive, Valence had great support from her husband and brother. While seeing her son so unresponsive was difficult, Valence knew she had to summon all of the faith she could, and had to have hope. She needed to be strong. Even when doctors told her that Robert might be a "vegetable," Valence didn't care. "I had faith in God that he was going to be okay, and I know my son. I could see something in his face that told me he would recover. I said to the doctor, 'No offense, but I'm going to trust in God. That's all I can do.' "

Valence visited Walter Reed's chapel that day to calm down and reflect on what happened to Robert. "That morning I went to the chapel to pray, but the individual room was occupied, so I went into the larger chapel. While I was praying I thought I heard a voice that said: 'Be still and know that I am God.' I got really scared, and ran out of the chapel, remembering what my mother always said: 'When you pray, you must be prepared to receive.' I think mentally I was not, and that's why I was scared. So for the rest of the day I did not speak to anyone."

As the doctors came in and out of Robert's room over the next few weeks, Valence was stressed out and always afraid that something would go terribly wrong. One day as she was about to enter his room, about seven o'clock in the morning, she saw the curtain drawn, and two nurses sitting next to his bed. They seemed nervous. She was so frightened. As she approached the room, the nurses told her she couldn't come in. Her heart sank. "What was happening to Robert?" Valence recalled thinking. "Was he even still alive?" About ten minutes later the nurses finally let her in. "As they pulled back the curtain, I heard Robert's voice for the first time. He said: 'Good morning, Ma.' I was crying, weeping, and I collapsed on the floor. I cried so hard. It was a miracle!"

Valence could not believe what had happened. Just as she expected the worst, her son spoke to her.

"I was so shocked. I called my husband right away and told him the good news. Robert was back." Not only could he speak, but she would eventually learn that Robert could also read and write. However, in the beginning, he couldn't walk, and he had very few motor skills and no short-term memory. Still, that was okay with Valence. "He was still here with us, and I considered it a blessing," Valence said.

As Robert began to recover, Valence gained strength from her family and faith, as well as from the other mothers she was beginning to get to know at Walter Reed. "This is such a horrible experience, but I was thankful that I was beginning to get some help and advice from the other moms who were facing the same traumas. We could share ideas about what was going on with our wounded warriors, and then be able to act on what we learned. For example, later on in Robert's recovery, we wanted to get him an appointment with a neuropsychiatrist, but they said it would take a couple of months. So another mom used her connections and was able to get that appointment for us in no time," said Valence.

Having the built-in support system would be a great comfort to Valence as she and Robert continued on their journey of recovery together.

Recovery for wounded warriors with TBIs is grueling. Every day is a struggle to regain some semblance of normalcy. Basic functions that many people take for granted are monumental tasks for TBI patients. In addition, the stress for the caregiver is off the charts, and Valence struggled every day as she tried to juggle her job with caring for Robert. Her husband needed to stay at home in Long Island. He needed to work, but he also couldn't emotionally handle seeing Robert in the condition he was in. "I love my husband, and we have a strong marriage, but he is a sensitive man, and I knew if he saw Robert in this state it would kill him. He didn't eat for weeks, and I had to call my neighbors at home to watch out for him."

Every day Valence was by Robert's side, only leaving the hospital to take a short nap or a shower. She traded places with her devoted brother, who stood by her side when Robert was first admitted to the hospital. By April, Robert was progressing nicely, and Valence got word that he would be transferred to the McGuire Veterans Affairs Hospital in Richmond, Virginia, where he would receive specialized care for his brain injury. He stayed there for three months, and his devoted mom was always nearby. In fact, every day at 5:00 a.m., Valence drove from her hotel in Richmond to the hospital before going to work in Washington, where her company had a satellite office, just so she could see that he was okay. "I wanted to see his face and just say 'good morning,' " Valence said. Relieved and comforted that Robert was still alive, she would do anything to make sure that his recovery progressed.

After a long workday in Washington, Valence drove back to Richmond. She would stop in Fredericksburg to pick up dinner for Robert, bring him the food, and stay with him until he finished eating. Then, she got back in her car and arrived at the hotel after midnight—only to do it all over again the next day. Sometimes, in order to make better time, Valence resorted to creating a fake passenger in her Honda Accord. She would take off her jacket and her hat and prop them up to look like there was someone in the vehicle with her. Luckily, the police never caught her driving in the HOV lane with a manufactured passenger. "Moms just do what they have to do," Valence said.

Though Robert continued to make progress, his recovery was complicated by personal issues that would eventually lead to him and Daphne getting a divorce. Once that struggle was over, though, Valence could focus heart and soul on what she knew would be a long and difficult road to recovery.

In July, Valence decided, along with Robert's medical team, to take him home for two months and spend time rehabilitating at Long Island Jewish Medical Center, which had a well-regarded day program. Since it was very close to home, Robert could spend time with his father, and they could all resume at least a brief semblance of family life. Valence and her extended family enjoyed having Robert around, and that was good for everyone's mental health. Following his time in New York, he was transferred to the military's brain center rehabilitation center in Johnstown, Pennsylvania, where Robert was expected to make further progress.

Valence made the long trip from New York to western Pennsylvania every weekend. She had to see her son. "Every Friday night I would drive seven hours to spend the weekend with Robert so he wouldn't have to be alone," Valence said. "I used to tell him that 'Mommy is going to be with you,' because I never wanted him to feel alone again. I could never get that image out of my mind. Imagining him by himself, worlds away from any family or friends—I couldn't ever let that happen to him again."

In 2011, the old Walter Reed medical complex to which Robert had returned following his stay in Pennsylvania was closing, and Robert, like all of the wounded warriors rehabilitating there, was transferred to the new Walter Reed National Military Medical Center in Bethesda, Maryland. It was there that Valence's bonds with the other Mighty Moms solidified. She knew, instinctively, that many of the women she had met at the old Walter Reed and the ones she would meet in the new medical center would become lifelong friends. Their children were her children. They were in this together.

Valence and Paulette Mason had already become fast friends, likewise Pam Britt and other moms, including Siobhan Fuller-McConnell and Tammy Karcher. Paulette and Tammy especially knew Valence's plight since their wounded warriors also suffered TBIs. "When you have friends like these moms who understand and care about you, it does give you strength, and they become your family," Valence said. "One time I was wearing this great dress, and Paulette told me how much she loved it. I said to myself that if I ever get out of here I'm going to find her that dress and give it to her as a gift."

Even with the supportive atmosphere and the progress that Robert had made, her son was not the man he used to be, and that troubled his mother. "My son was a really outgoing person, but after the brain injury he became quiet and withdrawn. Maybe he was a little depressed, too."

Even the simplest of tasks took time for Robert to process, and because he had no short-term memory, Valence had to remind him of literally everything.

Her day began this way: she would get up early, wake Robert up, and then prepare his breakfast. Once he was finished, she would tell him to take a shower, brush his teeth, and put on the clothing that she placed on his bed for the day. He would say, "Ma, I already took a shower," but just to be sure he would have to pass the smell test. "I would say, 'Robert, are you sure you took a shower?' and he said, 'Yes.' But when I got close to him I could tell that he just forgot, so I would gently remind him to go and do it again. Once he was clean and fed, she put him in the car and would drive fift miles to a vocational rehabilitation program that helped Robert learn th basic tasks he had all but forgotten. At the end of the day, Valence woul pick Robert up and then either take him out for dinner or go back and mak him the meal herself.

Fortunately, his rehabilitation therapists, some of the best in the busi ness, gave him a variety of games that he could play at home. They wer specially designed to increase his brain activity and keep his mind activ until he returned to therapy the next day.

"Robert had all kinds of therapeutic electronic games to play, and i also helped that we had a lot of family interaction," Valence added. "I the evenings the routine was a bit different, but we still had to work on hi short-term memory, and help him regain the most simple of tasks—evei knowing how to lace up his shoes." Valence said that Robert couldn't evei remember things he was told twenty minutes ago, though there was sligh improvement with short-term memory. "I am fortunate Robert and I hav such a close relationship because he feels comfortable with me taking car of him physically; but it is a daily challenge."

One example of those challenges was a story that Valence recountec during one of Robert's hospitalizations. "When he was in the hospital, h climbed out of his bed to get to the bathroom on his own, because he wa; embarrassed when the nurse would have to come to change the catheter. H said: 'Ma, can you do it?' Of course, I did, and I think having me around al the time really helped him get better much sooner."

Many of the moms have seen firsthand that wounded warriors who hav caring and engaged caregivers—moms, wives, dads, or others—are likely tc recover more quickly and psychologically adjust to their new lives much bet ter. "When I saw that Robert wanted to be alone, and was very low-key anc quiet, I knew I had to find out what was going on," said Valence. "Rober was definitely depressed, and I did everything I could during that time tc restore the family lifestyle that we had before."

Sometimes, too, Valence had to use her New York spunk to advocate on Robert's behalf. "One time the therapist told me that she was going tc give him a job on base, which we all thought was a great idea," said Valence "What I didn't know at the time was that they assigned him to work in the library. My son can't even find his way from the third floor of Building 62 to the first floor where the library was." As a result, Robert missed some days of work, and eventually, the physical therapy department made Valence aware of his poor performance by issuing a counseling statement—a written report with a negative warning by the squad leader that goes in a soldier's permanent record, may be given to the commander, and may result in disciplinary action. "I was furious," Valence said. "How can you give my son a job that requires him to do multiple tasks at once? Didn't anyone tell you my son has a brain injury?" Valence asked that the counseling statement be retracted, and the therapist apologized to her for assigning him that job in the first place.

"If you don't stand up for these soldiers, they just take them and put them anywhere," said Valence. "My son would be dead if I were not there. My son would have committed suicide. That's why I am always there for all of the wounded warriors here. It hurt me so badly one day when I saw another wounded warrior who had nobody with him. I would always try to reach out to talk to them as much as I could."

Another time, Valence demanded to see Robert's complete medical records. "I said that I wanted Robert's records to make sure his treatment was appropriate, and to check to see if he needed any other medical appointments. There was so much research on new treatments for brain injuries. I told them that if this was their child, they would want the best for them, too."

Even under normal circumstances, moms take care of their young like fierce lionesses. But, when those children are catastrophically injured during war, there is no stopping their roaring maternal instincts.

Day-to-day life for Robert and his mom remained a struggle. Valence lost her job after her company downsized, and without a job, and with Robert soon to be medically discharged, Valence was spent. Though she had great family support, her life as she knew it was gone. So many questions were in her mind. Would Robert ever be able to live on his own? Would she be able to return to New York? Would she ever work again? No one can appreciate how these Mighty Moms' lives are altered forever. They give up the most basic of life's pleasures, simple things like getting a haircut or manicure—not to mention not having the money they had before to buy a pair of new shoes or a special dress for a night out on the town. Nevertheless, Valence knew that she had to keep her spirits up to take care of Robert. "Every morning I got up and put on my makeup and did my hair," Valence said. "It was something that I could do that would make me feel good about myself."

Finally, on February 27, 2012, more than two years after his injury, Robert was medically discharged.

Fortunately, for Valence and other Mighty Moms, the nonprofit organization Operation Homefront came to the rescue by providing them with a townhouse in Gaithersburg, Maryland, not far from Washington, while Robert continued his rehabilitation. In addition to providing emergency funds, building smart homes for wounded warriors, and helping families of active duty service members and their families with a variety of much-needed services, they also help with free, temporary housing. Their "Operation Homefront Residences," located across the US, provide comfortable apartments along with support services from specially trained staff. "Operation Homefront helped me and Robert so much. Robert needed to be close to the things he was used to doing as well as his therapy," said Valence. "Plus, we had a built-in support network there, and Paulette and Pam and I were all there at the same time."

Robert continued to attend his vocational rehabilitation and was making progress, though he still had a long way to go. "Robert can't live 100 percent on his own," Valence added. "He is learning to do things more independently like putting gas in the car, or following GPS directions. I am trying to let him become more independent, and, finally, he can drive back and forth to his rehab, after almost two years of rehab. While it is hard to let go, I know I have to let him make mistakes. It is all part of the healing process."

One time, Valence recalls, Robert went to the gas station, but it took him a very long time to return. He was confused about the directions, but eventually figured it out, and that made Valence very happy. "It's so hard to retrain the brain, but Robert is really making progress. That's one of the reasons I think we will have to stay here for quite a while. He is so used to the routine, plus all of his rehabilitation is here. I guess my husband will have to deal with me being gone for a little more time. But, I don't have to worry about him at all. He's in the house by 9:30 p.m. every night, and he has to take care of the dog," she said jokingly.

One of the most heartwarming moments happened one weekend when Robert and Valence went for a trip to the Verizon store. She was looking at a phone case, complete with a battery charger, and she really wanted to buy it. "I loved that case, but thought spending $79 was too much. Robert said: 'Ma, I noticed you were looking at that case for a long time, and I want to buy it for you.' I said, 'That's okay, Robert, I don't really need it much anyway.' " About three days later, a package came in the mail from Verizon. It was the special case she wanted, sent to her by the most special man in her life.

Robert's decision to join the military and his subsequent traumatic brain injury were life-changing events for Valence, and the entire Scott family. For Robert, they were the source of a great deal of guilt. "Ma, I'm sorry to have put you and dad through this. I know dad wanted to retire, and you wanted to work, and didn't want you to give up your career," Robert said. Valence said, "I told him that 'it could have been me or Dad that got sick, and you would have to take care of us.' I wouldn't let him go there. I said, 'Robert, there are things in life that just happen. We are a family, and we always work together as a team.' " Robert just smiled.

Through it all, Robert never lost his strong will and his big heart, and he is positive about his future. "Hey, I'm a New Yorker. You have to suck it up and drive on; that's how we do it! On the positive side, I am still alive, and in the military you learn to never give up. Every day is a new day," Robert said. "I hope to work in the intelligence field or maybe work for the government," Robert added.

Robert gained some wisdom along the way, too, and said his mom is "the real deal" and is the "supermom of moms."

"My mom was always there for me," Robert said, "and guided me when I wasn't able to function on my own. She sacrificed so much for me, and helped me make the right decisions and get me to where I am today."

Valence told him, "Robert, parents always have wisdom, and God gave us an extra pair of wings and an extra pair of eyes to see beyond the horizon."

SEVEN

JEFFREY SHONK AND TAMMY KARCHER

AMMY KARCHER IS UNIQUE AMONG THE MOMS AT WALTER REED. SHE met the man who tried to kill her son, Jeffrey Shonk.

They met, Tammy and US Army Specialist Neftaly Platero, at his June 2012 trial for murder in a military courtroom at Fort Stewart, Georgia, about 6,750 miles from the base in Iraq where Platero killed two soldiers and wounded Jeffrey Shonk almost two years before.

Tammy wanted to confront the man responsible for her son's life-altering injuries. She wanted to ask, "Why would you do this?"

"This" was a shooting on September 23, 2010, just west of Baghdad, at Camp Fallujah, as the soldiers of the 3rd Battalion, 15th Infantry Regiment, 4th Infantry Brigade Combat Team, 3rd Infantry Division, were preparing to turn in for the night.

According to the press accounts, Private First Class Gebrah Noonan, of Watertown, Connecticut, had just returned from the showers to the room he shared with three others. Specialist John Carrillo Jr., of Stockton, California, was kneeling down, rummaging through his backpack. Jeffrey Shonk, of Maryland, was lying on his bunk, watching a movie on his computer. The military would later say that the four roommates had been arguing about keeping their room cleaned, but the "why" of what happened next may never be fully explained.

Platero drew his weapon and opened fire, eighteen times in all. Noonan, twenty-six, was hit in the side and the back. Twenty-year-old Carrillo, who

109

was married with two children, one a newborn when he deployed just two months earlier, was shot in the back seven times. Private First Class Shonk, then twenty-one, was shot in the left leg, the right hand, and the head. Neither Noonan nor Carrillo survived his wounds. It wasn't immediately clear if Shonk would either.

"Why would you do this? That was my biggest thing," Tammy said years later, still in disbelief. "Why turn the gun on your brothers?"

It was an unfathomable thought for Tammy, whose father, George Glenn, had served as a Green Beret in Vietnam, and whose husband had been a career Navy man. She knew the bonds service members had with each other, and had seen it most dramatically when her father attended Jeffrey's basic training graduation. It was one of the few times she'd seen her father cry. As anyone in the military knows, risks come with the job. Military families understand this. Threats from the enemy in times of war are a constant source of worry. But from one of your own? Part of your extended military family?

Tammy's extended family, what she calls her "friends for life," began developing years ago. Some date back to when Jeffrey was born in Carthage, New York, near Fort Drum, where his father, Tammy's first husband, was stationed. Two of those friends, Terry and Barb, shared Thanksgiving and Christmas with Tammy and her family, and they later became godparents to Jeffrey. In fact, as Tammy said, "They got to see him before my family did." They stayed close, and there were many other close friends along the way. Tammy's second husband, Tom, was a career Navy man, so her extended military family continued to grow, through tours that took them to Sicily twice, and three times to Maryland, where Jeffrey would sign up for the Army during his senior year of high school.

It was no surprise then that Tammy reached out to parts of that military family in the difficult, confusing time after she learned that Jeffrey was hurt, but before she could lay eyes on him and provide some comfort. At that moment, she was the one in need of comfort.

"When I first got the call, I knew what questions to ask, but my mind was with my son," Tammy recalled. "I told them they'd have to talk to my husband. He'd have a clear head. I was totally freaked. My heart was in my toes. I was worried. Is he going to make it? I couldn't get to him."

Waiting for Tom to get home from work, and with her wounded son thousands of miles away, Tammy felt helpless. She knew he had been hurt.

She knew that the injuries were serious. But, in the shock of the moment, she hadn't been able to absorb details. She couldn't stop thinking the worst.

"A lot of unknowns were the issue, the what-ifs," Tammy remembers. "Would I have to care for my child for the rest of his life? Or care for him at home or in a nursing home? Was I going to walk into his room and see a vegetable? All these things were running through my mind."

In the meantime, she called her family in Ohio, making sure to talk to her sister rather than upset her elderly parents. She also contacted Jeffrey's friends at Fort Stewart, Georgia, home base for the Third Infantry Division. Tammy thought that the other families of soldiers in Jeffrey's unit might have more news. She had been hearing from him regularly up until a few days before he was wounded. Because he was a communications specialist, she thought he was in a "safe zone," not out in the field where he could be wounded. But friends in Georgia had no information to relieve her anguish.

Later that day, Tammy was on the front porch, smoking a cigarette and being comforted by neighbors—more retired military—when her husband Tom came outside after taking a follow-up call about Jeffrey.

"The look on his face," Tammy said, pausing. "I'm gonna choke up. It always happens when I talk about this."

She asked him what was wrong.

"A fellow soldier shot our son," Tom said. "What did that mean?" she asked him, still not understanding what had happened. "It means that one of our own turned on Jeffrey," he replied.

Again, there were few details. Of course, the Army had just started its own investigation. Officials didn't have all the answers themselves, and they were careful not to pass along anything that would jeopardize a subsequent prosecution. The family did not know at that point the who or why of the attack on Jeffrey. They didn't know that others had been killed. And only gradually did they learn, from subsequent telephone calls, how Jeffrey was doing. In one call his condition would be described as "stable." Then, in another, "critical." Then "grave." During a late-night call on the day she learned about the attack, Tammy found out that Jeffrey had a tracheotomy, and his head wound was being described as a "grazing." "But I didn't understand what grazing meant," Tammy said.

Jeffrey had suffered two serious wounds. The most life-threatening was his head wound. Jeffrey had been lying on his bunk, watching a movie on his laptop, and was facing Platero when he was shot. The bullet aimed at his head grazed his skull about an inch above the hairline, leaving a three inch wound that didn't penetrate the skull but rattled his head, later caus ing brain swelling and a severe TBI. The second serious wound was in hi lower left leg, where the bullet had blown off about four inches of his tibi and cracked the fibula in two places. His leg bled so badly that when hel] arrived, within minutes of the shooting, they thought he was dead. His thir wound was in his hand, which was hit as he instinctively lifted it to protec himself.

Three days later, a Sunday, Tammy was talking to the neurosurgeon wh was looking after her son about the head wound. "He kept telling me abou Jeffrey's intracranial pressure levels, called ICPs," Tammy said. "He kep telling me they were from twenty-five to forty-five. I didn't understand wha that meant."

ICP levels measure the pressure of the cerebrospinal fluid in the spac between the skull and the brain. There are different ways to monitor ICI levels, but the one used in Jeffrey's case involved inserting a hollow subdura screw through a hole drilled into the skull, which then allows the sensor t record from inside the subdural space. ICPs are measured in millimeters o mercury (mm Hg), with the normal range for an adult being 7 to 15 mm Hg Elevated levels are often seen in the event of head trauma, with anythin; over 20 mm Hg considered dangerous. If not recognized and if the pres sure is not relieved, the abnormally high levels can cause severe neurologica damage or be fatal.

Initially, doctors had hoped that Jeffrey, who had been transported from Iraq to the Landstuhl hospital in Germany, would be stable enough to be sent back to the States by Tuesday, five days after the shooting. However even in the darkened intensive care unit, the slightest movement or faintes light was causing his ICP levels to spike. The decision was made to keep Jef frey in Germany, and bring his family—Tammy, Tom, and Jeffrey's sixteen year-old sister, Kourtnee—to him.

"As we went over, he was still in critical condition," Tammy said. "I wa: taking Benadryl so I could sleep on the plane. When I got there I wanted t be totally focused on him, giving him positive energy. I wanted to let hin know that we were there and that he had to fight."

She still had many questions about the shooting, including whether he son had done something to cause it. "I had a lot of time to think, too mucl time, and I didn't have any idea what was going on," she said. A call over th weekend with an Army colonel had dispelled some of the mystery. He told Tammy that the shooter had been apprehended and that two other soldiers had been killed. "My heart sank," Tammy recalled.

Upon their arrival in Germany on Wednesday morning, Tammy wanted the family checked into their quarters, showered, and fed before seeing Jeffrey. If there was any paperwork to do, she wanted it out of the way beforehand. Once she was with him, she wanted no distractions. He would have her undivided attention.

"We got upstairs to the ICU area about two o'clock, and they took us into the little chapel, my husband, my daughter, and me," Tammy said. "They had the chaplain with us as well, in case we needed him to prepare us for what we were going to see.

"My dad had been real sick when I was eighteen, and he looked like the inside of a radio with all the wires and tons of everything around. So I knew what I was walking into that day, but I didn't know the severity."

Before they entered, the neurosurgeon and another doctor explained all the machines in the room, the fourteen IVs hooked up to Jeffrey, and the fact that he was in a medically induced coma. Then they walked the family inside. The lights were off. Nurses were gentle and quiet when moving him or adjusting anything. The slightest noise, or stirring, could cause his ICP levels to rise dramatically.

"Jeffrey looked like he had gained one hundred pounds, all from swelling," Tammy said. "There were no wrinkles in his knuckles. His head was all wrapped up."

The doctors explained how the bullet had shaken his brain, but didn't penetrate the skull. Miraculously, it hadn't even caused a fracture.

"You think it would have, but didn't," Tammy thought at the time. "He must've had an angel sitting on his shoulder."

He did, in a sense. Her father, the onetime Green Beret, had given Jeffrey a clear rock with an angel in it before his deployment. "I don't know what it means, but my dad said to carry it with him at all times," Tammy said. "My son joined the military to follow in Dad's footsteps. He was the first grandbaby, so Dad and he have a very tight bond."

The three of them remained with Jeffrey until about ten o'clock that evening, when Tom and Kourtnee decided to return to the Fisher House, where they would be staying while in Germany. Tammy, however, wasn't going anywhere.

"I was not leaving," Tammy said. "My husband knew that I wasn't. I stayed at the ICU. I made sure it was okay with the doctors, and they said it wasn't a problem. But it was so touch and go."

Throughout those first hours, the doctors made clear the danger of the spiking ICP levels. There were signs of improvement, but not enough to prevent brain damage. If Jeffrey's condition didn't change within twenty-four hours, they warned, they would have to operate, removing the left part of his head in an attempt to relieve the pressure. That's exactly what happened. Tammy was there when they came for Jeffrey at 6:00 a.m. for the three-and-a-half-hour surgery. It was September 30, one week after the shooting.

"That day he was doing okay," Tammy said of his condition after the procedure. "The ICP levels were back and forth, up and down, because of all the sedation and everything. But finally they got down to twenty. I think that was two days later, and the doctors said, 'We can deal with that. But we don't want them up to thirty-five and forty again.'"

She started to believe her son was going to be all right. Another encouraging sign came shortly thereafter.

"One day he opened his eye for me," Tammy said. "Only the one. I got to see that big blue eye. It was like he was born again."

Somewhere inside, beyond the tubes and monitors and bandages, her son was still there. And, finally, his condition was stabilizing enough so that doctors could think about sending him back to the States.

At Landstuhl, Tammy had regularly been reminded that her son was not alone in dealing with injuries from the War on Terror. When she stepped outside for a cigarette, she was usually near the emergency room, which was right where the newly wounded were brought from the airfield. However, when a new group was scheduled to arrive, Tammy was warned by a security guard to stay away for a couple of hours. "He knew I didn't want to see them being brought in," Tammy said. "It was too heart wrenching."

She could get an idea of how many traumatically injured soldiers were coming by the number of waiting beds lined up outside the ER doors—often dozens. She didn't actually see a blue ambulance bus until after more than a week at Landstuhl. It was the one that would take would take Jeffrey to the airfield for his trip home. The family would return on a separate flight, but before being separated, Tammy sat with Jeffrey on his bus until it was ready to pull away. "They let me stay with him," Tammy said thankfully.

The separation wasn't for very long. The family touched down in Washington, DC, and checked into a hotel, and Tammy was reunited with Jeffrey in the ICU by seven thirty that night, at what was known as Bethesda Naval Hospital (now part of the Walter Reed National Military Medical Center).

He would spend three and a half weeks in the ICU, and there began the next phase of a lengthy and grueling recovery, coming out of the medically induced coma and being removed from the ventilator. The first week after being revived was a blur, for Jeffrey especially. His first memory after waking up was of visiting family, but in fact they didn't arrive until he had been awake for ten days. While there was joy in having him back—Tammy said he was laughing and writing different things from the start, none of which he remembers—there were also fears. "We didn't know if he would walk or talk again," Tammy said. "We didn't know if there was brain damage. We didn't know where he would be."

He would eventually be up and about, but only after countless hours of therapy and about four dozen surgeries to repair his lower leg. The damage to the frontal lobe of his brain, the area that helps regulate decision making, problem solving, behavior control, consciousness, and emotions, was not as bad as they first feared, but there were issues, some of which continue.

Tammy describes his state upon first waking from the coma as that of a two-year-old. He was still woozy, and it was easy to distract him.

"They really didn't know how well he'd be because of the frontal lobe damage," Tammy said. "Age has lots to do with it. The brain doesn't really stop developing until about age twenty-six, so his brain is still developing. And each person is different. You just don't know what the outcome will be or how well each body can fight to regain anything."

As with many TBI victims, Jeffrey struggles with memory, impulse control, and regulating his emotions.

"To this day, we have issues with emotions," Tammy said. "It's like a light switch."

Any incident can trigger sudden and dramatic changes in Jeffrey's mood and behavior, even something as common as pulling in front of him while he's driving. Erratic and unpredictable actions are also common with a traumatic brain injury, and Jeffrey can have trouble with impulse control, which means he'll sometimes say "inappropriate things," according to his mom.

"If he starts talking out, I have to redirect him and say, 'No, you shouldn' talk like that,' " Tammy said. "But, he's also twenty-four, so I have to pick and choose my battles with him."

Jeffrey can be aware of the behaviors to a certain extent, but he is often unable to control them. "He has good days and bad days," Tammy said "You can tell how he'll be when he wakes up, depending how much sleep he gets. The more, the better. In some ways he's like a toddler. If he doesn' get enough sleep, he's cranky all day. Not enough sleep, and anything can trigger him."

His mom knows him all too well and often can see the triggers before an outburst. In one early therapy session, Jeffrey was asked to build a chair with different pieces of PVC pipe. He had no written instructions, but was required to answer a phone every few minutes and take notes from the caller. Despite the distraction of a constantly ringing phone, he had to follow the caller's instructions to complete the chair—all with a deadline.

"I think it was a ten- to twelve-minute exercise," Tammy recalls. "Three minutes into it, I could see he was getting aggravated. I can read my son."

The therapy sessions were a way to awaken information inside his brain, to retrain him, starting at a prekindergarten level in many respects. The staff used basic memory and trivia games, as well as speech therapies, all designed to improve his retention of information. "They had to wake his mind back up," Tammy said. Sometimes Tammy didn't attend the sessions, because the therapists didn't want Jeffrey turning to her for answers. They wanted him to be more independent. Other times she'd find herself just as frustrated by the exercise as her son was. They would start with easy questions. What is your full name? What's your birth date? What month is it? Who's the president? But then they might ask to name the months that have thirty-one days

Jeffrey uses a variety of tools to help him remember things, including iPads, calendars, and a small spiral notebook that he keeps in his chest pocket. "Every little thing that you and I take for granted, we have to retrain for Jeffrey," Tammy said.

"He's better now than he was," said his mom. "But a brain injury can take up to two years to heal. Usually the first year, you know what you're going to get. If you use the right therapies, you can get through and work that portion of the brain to get it to the best it's going to be."

All the while, he also needed physical therapy to recover from his leg wound. Back in Germany, doctors had begun the repair process, with surgery every other day even while he was still in a coma. Jeffrey had been given a stabilizer bar, essentially a piece of metal attached to the bones by pins to keep the leg stable, on September 24. Once in the States, he had physical therapy twice a day on Mondays, Wednesdays, and Fridays.

At first, Tammy said, therapy meant getting him out of bed, putting him in a wheelchair, and wheeling him around the physical therapy room a few times. Even that was exhausting. "He was real frail at the beginning," Tammy said. "He didn't even get out of the chair. He just rode around." Other days they might let him stay in bed and work his legs from there. Then it was back to moving him from bed to wheelchair and back again, and he'd be utterly exhausted. He looked it, too. That once swelled-up young man whom Tammy had first seen in Germany was down to about one hundred pounds—from his normal weight of 175. "He looked like an eighty- to ninety-year-old man," his mom said. "He was just basically skin and bones."

His stabilizer bar was replaced in early November with an external fix-ator, a frame with three rings—one right below the knee, one at the middle of the tibia, and one toward the ankle—that was attached to the leg with wires and pins. He kept that on, by Tammy's count, for eleven months and two days. "That's what was on while he learned to walk again," Tammy said. That process began at the beginning of December, when Jeffrey started to use crutches. While his leg bone was regrowing—replacing the part that was shot away—it was Tammy's job to adjust the struts on the external fixator, which she did for one hundred days. By February, the bone was pushing on the antibiotic beads that had been placed in the wound early on. He underwent surgery again to remove the beads and insert a piece of synthetic bone to fuse with his real bone. It would be another month before he could apply pressure on his leg.

Even the issue of smoking was raised as part of the healing process. He had started to smoke while in the service, and doctors told him that the habit could affect blood flow in the tiny capillaries in his leg. If he didn't stop, they warned, he could lose the leg. He took their advice for about eighteen months, according to his mom. She had once planned to kick her own habit by November 2010, before Jeffrey came home for Thanksgiving on R&R. It was something her kids had always bugged her about. "I wanted to be through the bitchy stage by the time he came home," Tammy recalls. "I wanted to show him I could do it." His shooting that September changed her plan. "I'm too stressed to even think about quitting," Tammy said.

There was stress and then some. She not only went through the trauma of seeing her only son grievously wounded, but she was also there with emotional support for him from the moment she stepped into the ICU in Germany. Furthermore, like many of the moms at Walter Reed, she was her son's nurse, his liaison with medical staff, and the one who scheduled appointments (and saw to it that he kept them) and ordered medications. She stepped back in therapy sessions, even when it hurt her, so he wouldn't use her as a crutch.

In the process, Tammy lost her job.

Since October 2006, she had been a civilian employee of a contractor at Naval Air Station Patuxent River in Maryland. To care for Jeffrey, she used the time she was eligible for under the federal Family and Medical Leave Act, even extending it by working from the hospital or returning to the office for short stints. However, by August 2011, she was fired. The company needed a full-time employee. Tammy understood but said she was "very hurt." Still, she had no choice. Jeffrey needed a full-time caretaker.

And there was yet one more burden she carried, unknown to Jeffrey. In fact, part of the difficulty for her was keeping any knowledge of it from him.

While Jeffrey healed, the legal process that began right after the shooting in Camp Fallujah proceeded. In that phone call with the Army colonel before she traveled to Germany, Tammy was explicitly asked not to speak to her son about what happened to him. The US Army's Criminal Investigation Command (abbreviated as CID, for Criminal Investigation Division) wanted to talk to him first. They didn't want the family inadvertently passing along misinformation that might somehow cloud what Jeffrey—the only surviving witness to the attack—would be able to remember, if anything.

"For a long time I lied to my son," Tammy said. "When he first woke up, he didn't really know what happened, he didn't know where he was. He knew he was in the hospital. 'You've been shot,' was all I said. Because I couldn't tell him until the agents got hold of him." At that point, still dazed and confused from coming out of the coma, he didn't ask questions, and if he did he was easy to distract.

If anyone called about the case, whether CID, the Navy Criminal Investigative Service, the prosecutors, or someone from Jeffrey's unit, Tammy excused herself and took the call in the hallway. When an NCIS agent was prepared to walk the family through the process, and answer any questions, they found another room for the discussion, leaving Tammy's dad with Jeffrey.

The agent explained the differences between civilian and military court proceedings. The Article 32 proceeding was the equivalent of a preliminary hearing, the name taken from Article 32 of the United States Uniform Code of Military Justice. The court-martial would be the trial. There would be a judge (an officer) and a jury (in this case five service members, commissioned and noncommissioned). NCIS would need all of Jeffrey's medical records. And soon, when he was up to it, they would be coming to him for print and DNA evidence. The agent explained that they were sorting through the evidence found in the room where the shootings had occurred and were determining what prints or blood samples belonged to which soldier.

Jeffrey found out about Noonan and Carrillo on November 9. He was talking to a noncommissioned officer from his unit, with whom he was close, and he asked how his two roommates were. The sergeant didn't tell Jeffrey what happened, but he did say that the two soldiers didn't make it. "Of course, he cried," Tammy said. "He didn't understand. And then he asked if Platero was dead or alive, and they just said he was incarcerated."

Collecting Jeffrey's prints turned out to be a break in the routine. "After watching *CSI* and seeing all that on TV, it was pretty cool seeing the other side," Tammy admits. They took prints of his fingers, his fist, and his hand, the last by inking his palm and having him grasp a bottle with paper wrapped around it. Jeffrey found it all "pretty cool," his mom said, but he did have questions afterward. "He understood, but he didn't understand," Tammy said. "He wasn't fully there."

When the agents came by to talk, Jeffrey's doctor would sit in, monitoring his patient's emotions. They didn't want him agitated, and would only allow the agents to talk to him for ten minutes at a time. He was having daily headaches at that point, and too much stimulation brought on the pain. "They didn't want to push him too much," Tammy recalled.

The Article 32 was originally scheduled for around Thanksgiving, but was delayed a month . . . and then another . . . and then one more. It was eventually done by teleconference, in a secure room over a secure line, because the defendant was still in Iraq. Tammy entered the room with Jeffrey, but was asked to leave. Shortly after, Jeffrey emerged, agitated. They had asked questions he wasn't prepared to answer. So then, unexpectedly,

Tammy was asked to testify. "The attorneys didn't tell me that I'd have to speak, so I felt like I was thrown under the bus and was very aggravated," Tammy said. "I'm not part of this. I'm the mom. I'm the caregiver. I was really agitated." The lawyers called her back that evening to explain. During his testimony, Jeffrey had said something they didn't understand, something he reported had been told to him but he misunderstood. They had hoped Tammy would clarify it for them.

After that, anything related to the case upset Jeffrey. "Every time he got back into his groove, as he was becoming my Jeffrey again, something would happen, and he'd be back in that state, and his anxiety would surface," Tammy recalls.

The bottom line was that Jeffrey couldn't remember what happened in the room the night of the shooting. Yet the lawyers and others involved in the case kept coming back. "I think we talked fifteen, twenty times in person," Tammy said. "They always came to see us. We never went to see them. Because, for one, Jeffrey couldn't fly."

Tammy and Jeffrey did travel to Georgia in June, spending almost three weeks there visiting with members of his unit. "He did really well," Tammy recalled. The trip included a stop at Fort Stewart's Warriors Walk, a memorial grove with more than 460 trees, each one planted in honor of a member of the 3rd Division killed in Afghanistan or Iraq since 2003.

Within days after the Article 32, Platero was returned to the States, and further proceedings would be at their unit's home base, Fort Stewart. The stress during the ensuing weeks, especially the stretch from late summer through the fall, was particularly grueling. At one point, Jeffrey was needed for a phone-call hearing to determine whether to seek the death penalty against Platero. The family was also dealing with a move necessitated by the merger of Bethesda and Walter Reed. And Jeffrey's leg became infected, not once but twice. Even the one bright spot of that time, the removal of the external fixator because the leg bone was hard enough, still required some adjustment.

"He was not dealing with things well," Tammy said. "There was a lot going on in those six to eight weeks. He was agitated, confused. He wasn't sleeping, and was aggressive. Depression set in, and it was really bad."

The court-martial was set for November, then December, and then January. "They kept asking for a continuance," Tammy said. "They weren't ready, they weren't ready, and they weren't ready."

And in the midst of all that, during a December hearing, Jeffrey's name was released to the media for the first time. Tammy had tried hard to keep this from happening, at least until the trial. As the legal proceedings dragged on, she didn't want news crews bothering her, her son, or her extended family. "I was livid," Tammy said. "I was so mad. They didn't forewarn me or anything."

The wounded, she argues, never make the news, unless it's reported in a small-town paper. "The media only lets you know about those who have died," Tammy said. "So many are injured, but you never hear about them."

The release, amid so much else, was just one thing too many.

"So not only am I dealing with Jeffrey's day-to-day injuries, and being his caregiver, but I had the trial and the lawyers, and the whole nine-yard stress," Tammy said.

Tammy knows that, in one sense, she is fortunate. Her son came home, while too many others did not. "Yes, I have my son," she said. "But he's not the son I sent to war. My son has been tampered with. So I have to deal with the new Jeffrey. And that is the hardest part, because I'm still dealing with it."

Finally, the trial was scheduled to begin in June. Jeffrey planned to drive, though his mother wasn't thrilled with the idea. But the trial was expected to last about three weeks, and the family was warned that cross-examinations can take time. He wanted the freedom of having his own car while spending all that time in Georgia. It was decided that he would travel with the niece of a family friend—part of that extended military family. She was interested in the law, and she knew Jeffrey well, so Tammy thought she'd be able to help keep him calm, and perhaps lighten his mood as the trial raised tensions for them all.

Tammy flew, and Tom planned to drive down later. He didn't want to take too much time off work, but Tammy knew she'd need him there at some point. That point came much quicker than expected. Despite the pre-trial delays, and the dozens and dozens of witnesses called at the Article 32, the court-martial moved along briskly.

In the end, it would last just over a week, and Tammy remembers each day as being stressful. "The first day was very hard," Tammy said. "Seeing everything was overwhelming." At the same time, being there helped fill in so many blanks for her. She was able to talk to the doctor who had cared for Jeffrey in Iraq and the medic who'd arrived first on the scene. She learned how Camp Fallujah was laid out. She saw pictures of the crime scene. And she met the families of the two soldiers who were killed.

When the defense first called for a mistrial, Tammy's heart dropped. Would the court-martial be over before it had begun? But officials explained this was a pro forma request, one that would be repeated several times. And the request was rejected each time it was made.

For Tammy, one part of the experience stood out: "It was the first time I got to see the killer."

"I had seen pictures," Tammy said, "but to come face-to-face with the person who tried to kill my son was . . ." Her voice trailed off. "I wanted to look him in the face. I really wanted to talk to him, but couldn't. I wanted to say, 'Why? Why would you do this? … Why turn your gun on your brothers?'"

The "why" never came. Platero didn't testify, though his attorney talked about a letter his client had written. But Tammy noted that the letter "never said he was sorry. He saw the pain he caused his family and other families involved, but he never said he was sorry."

Jeffrey wasn't allowed in the courtroom until his own testimony. Before he entered, his mother worried about how he would react to seeing Platero for the first time since the shootings. The defendant was seated only five feet from the witness stand.

"We didn't want Jeffrey to talk out when he wasn't supposed to," Tammy said. "We didn't know what emotions might come over him."

When she raised her concerns with the lawyers, they moved Platero from the end of the table to the center, in between his lawyers. Jeffrey was walked to the stand by an attorney, who made a point of keeping himself between Jeffrey and the table where Platero sat. Jeffrey was using a cane. At that point he had become more used to walking again, though usually in tennis shoes. This was his first time back in full uniform, including dress shoes. His mother urged him to use the cane, to keep steady on his feet, and for something to lean on should anxiety strike.

Tammy remembers him being asked his name, his rank, his social security number. Where was he stationed? Had he been in Fallujah? Then, do you know who shot you? Do you remember being shot? "I was on pins and needles, for fear of what he'd say," Tammy said. But he simply answered, "No."

His mother couldn't have been more relieved when that phase of the trial was over. "He did really well. I thought he held it together."

The jury was out for only ninety minutes. When they returned, Platero was found guilty of two counts of premeditated murder and one count of attempted premeditated murder. Because a decision had been made at an earlier hearing not to pursue the death penalty, the sentencing phase that came next had only to decide if Platero would be given life with or without the possibility of parole.

Tammy was called to testify, and one of the first questions she was asked was how she felt about sending a son to war. She believes her answer shocked the panel. "I'm not a real religious person," Tammy recalled saying, "but regardless of where you're at, whether driving down the road or walking down the street, if it's his time to go, it's his time to go. There's nothing I can do about that. But never, in my wildest dreams, did I ever believe that his brother in arms would try to kill him. I knew the enemy might shoot at him, but never thought his own brother in arms would."

Then she described the life that she and Jeffrey had been leading since September 23, 2010. How many appointments he had each week, how many physical therapies, how many surgeries. She described the model of Jeffrey's head that she'd been shown when he had his brain surgery, and the titanium plate that replaced the piece of skull that had been removed to save his life.

"Will your son ever be the same?" Tammy was asked. "No, he'll always have to have access to care, 24-7. He may remember conversations, he may not. He has good days and bad days." What was a day like? She described cleaning the pins on his leg. She talked about being away from home, what she'd had to miss. She'd been away when Kourtnee got her driver's license, when she'd attended her first day of tech school, and later her first day of college. "I missed the most important years of a teen's life," Tammy said, "because I chose to be with my son, to take care of him."

Tammy was nervous while on the stand, but said she made a point of looking directly at the jury. She tried to read their minds by the looks on their faces, and believes at least one teared up during her testimony.

Jeffrey followed her to the stand. He was shown pictures, one of his boot camp graduation, and another of him and his grandfather. He was asked to talk about what he was feeling those days, and why he chose to go into the military. Then he was shown a picture from before boot camp. It was a family portrait that Tammy had insisted on having taken before her son went away. It showed her, Jeffrey, and Kourtnee. When asked to explain who was in the photo, Jeffrey started to cry.

"Why the tears?" he was asked.

"Because I'll never look like that again."

It took about an hour for the jury to sentence Platero to life without parole, a decision that was automatically appealed to the Army Court of Criminal Appeals.

Much later, Tammy would recall a conversation that a Marine first sergeant had with some of her friends—yes, from that extended military family, which now includes the moms of Walter Reed. He tried to tell them what to expect when their sons returned from war. "He may be the same, and he may be different," he told them.

No one understands that better than Tammy. She is blessed that Jeffrey came home, the same sweet, loving, and sometimes irascible young man who went away. She is hopeful as she watches him regain his independence, securing an internship with the NAVAIR Wounded Warrior Program and renting an apartment. But he is different. Tammy, too. She is the same loving, fiercely protective mom who sent her son off to war. But she, like Jeffrey, has also become a warrior, fighting alongside her son as he makes his way in the world.

EIGHT

ADAM KEYS AND JULIE KEYS

JULIE KEYS HAS GRACE. THAT PARADOXICAL QUALITY ALLOWS SOMEONE TO not crack under pressure, handle the most difficult situations with dignity and poise, and most of all, sacrifice her emotional needs for a greater purpose. Tall and elegant, with hazel eyes that shine with compassion, Julie has grace in spades. From the first moment she learned her son, Adam, was critically injured in July 2010, after a roadside bomb killed four of his teammates, including his best friend, to helping him through nearly 140 surgeries, Julie has earned her Mighty Mom medals. And grace is a quality that runs in the family. Both Julie and Adam, a young war hero who has survived unimaginable circumstances, are strong, determined, affable, and optimistic.

Though Julie, fifty-four, was born in Nova Scotia, Canada, she has lived in the United States for more than twenty years, in Whitehall, Pennsylvania. Except for a few classic Canadian pronunciations of words such as "out" and "about," she is as American as it gets. She loves parades, the *New York Times* crossword puzzle, a good cup of coffee, and of course, the US Army. She and her husband, Stephen, have been married for thirty-two years, and currently, Julie lives in Bethesda with Adam. Stephen lived in Fort Myers, Florida, where he moved for his job, but he moved to Bethesda in the spring. In addition to Adam, they have a daughter, Courtney, who is in California with her husband, Benjamin, and the Keys's new grandson, born in December 2013. Julie's life was going really well. She enjoyed her job working in a medical lab, she had a solid and happy marriage, and both of her children were happy, healthy young adults.

When Adam decided to enlist in the US Army, along with his best friend, Jesse Reed, Julie was nervous. But she knew this was what Adam wanted, and when he put his mind to something, there was no doubt that he would be the best. He told Julie, "It's my dream, and if I don't do it now I will regret it for the rest of my life."

Two weeks before leaving for Fort Bragg to complete his one-month training period before deploying to Afghanistan, Adam married Rosie, a young woman he had been dating on and off for about four years.

Then, on July 14, 2010, Julie and her family's lives would take an unexpected turn for the worse. She would need to call upon as much grace and strength as she could muster.

Seven months into Adam's deployment, Julie was having lunch with a friend when she received a call from her husband. "Stephen said he had something to tell me, and asked me if I wanted to hear it on the phone or wait until I got home," Julie said. "I said, 'Tell me now,' and he told me the horrible news that Jesse, Adam's best friend, had been killed in action. Rosie called me when I was on my way home, and she met me at my house. I knew Adam was with Jesse, but since we didn't hear anything about him, I assumed that was good news. But I was still so scared."

"I knew that if something did happen to Adam that they would call us," Julie said. Julie and Rosie were literally pacing around the house and decided to go to the local firehouse where they knew they would get support, since that was the place Adam and the rest of the family would frequent. They had a lot of friends there, and Julie said that did provide some comfort. However, when they finally returned home, there was still no word about Adam.

"I just needed to hear something. I was up all night and kept getting up every couple of hours to check the computer to see if we got any emails. In the morning I picked up Rosie, and she came to stay with us at our house."

Then, at 7:00 a.m. Rosie's phone rang. It was someone from Fort Bragg. "They told me that Adam had been injured, and she passed the phone to me. They said: 'Mrs. Keys, your son, Adam, was critically injured.' "

"The man on the other end of the phone was very nice. He told me to take down his number, and that when I calmed down, I could call him back. He said to write all of my questions down on paper, and he could answer them once I had a chance to take it all in. My first question was, 'Does he have all of his arms and legs?' He told me he did, and then began to list all of Adam's injuries, starting from the head down," said Julie. "He told me that Adam would be medevaced to Germany, where they were going to stabilize him, but he would need an operation first at the hospital in Kandahar. He had a severe brain injury, many broken bones in his shoulder and both legs, severe trauma to his face, and eye injuries. The good news was that he was in critical but stable condition. Strangely they were good words to hear. At least Adam was alive."

Adam, Jesse, and their fellow soldiers, Chase, Matt, and Zach, had been riding in a RG31 armored vehicle, the second vehicle in a convoy that had stopped to sweep for IEDs. There had recently been a severe sandstorm, which made the IEDs more difficult to detect. During a sandstorm, and with no air support, the terrorists have more time to place larger IEDs, and the soldiers knew this at the outset.

Even with all the preplanning and caution used in sweeping for IEDs, still, one was unexpectedly detonated remotely. It struck with such force that Adam's vehicle was literally airborne. The soldiers in the third vehicle recalled seeing it blown straight up in the air, then crashing down with unimaginable force.

After Julie calmed down from the news she had just heard, she decided to call the Department of the Army to ask if she should fly to Germany to be with Adam. They said he was stable, and would be on the next available transport to the US. "He had to wait six days because all of the transports were full," Julie said. "They were really good to us, and were patient with us calling Germany many, many times a day to check on Adam's condition. They had him in a medically induced coma—a procedure that would help expedite the healing process. They also made sure our transport coincided with Adam's, so we were very grateful for that."

Julie and her family couldn't wait to see Adam again.

It didn't matter to them what shape he was in, or what he looked like. They were just happy he was alive. "When we went into the room there were so many tubes and wires everywhere. It was like we knew it was really bad, and it was terrible seeing Adam hooked up to all of those monitors. I thought that while this is really bad and scary, it is very fixable; he was still in one piece," Julie said. "Adam was hooked up to so many things, but we still knew it was him, even with the tubes and this Bair Hugger contraption that wraps around him and helps regulate his temperature. They were giving him broad-spectrum antibiotics. We thought he seemed okay."

Julie said that throughout the day, the nurses and doctors would come in, stop the sedation to see if he would wake up enough to respond to questions and commands, and ask him to wiggle his toes or squeeze their fingers. On Saturday Adam's fever started to abate, and Julie felt a bit of relief. But that, sadly, was to be short-lived.

Adam was scheduled for surgery on his broken bones Monday morning. On Sunday, an infection went septic throughout his bloodstream. He continued to get worse as each hour passed, and Julie was horrified to see Adam—her handsome, though beaten-up, son—become so swollen and so sick. Julie said his body looked just like the Michelin Man. She had never seen anything like this before in her life. Julie was staying with Adam that night. About 8:30 p.m. the doctors were scurrying around, and she knew something was really wrong. "I didn't know what was going on," Julie said, clearly anguished.

Julie overheard the doctors saying they needed to operate on Adam that night. "They said they had to take him to the operating room because they needed to go in and see where the infection was coming from. They said that if it were in his intestine, it would be 'incompatible with life.' I was standing there going, 'What?' One of the doctors then told us that we needed to give him permission to do the surgery, but I couldn't relay this to my family because I was so distraught."

Thankfully for Adam, the infection wasn't in his intestine, but the doctors did have to open up his belly to relieve all of the pressure and, hopefully, reduce the grotesque swelling.

Unfortunately, things just went from bad to worse. "Because of the infection they had to put Adam on blood pressure suppressors to keep his heart and brain functioning, which in turn lessened the blood flow to his extremities. Because his skin had blown up so much, it literally began to peel off. We could actually see his skin turning brown; it was like watching his limbs just melt away," Julie said. "The doctors told us that the cocktail of antibiotics that Adam was taking may or may not work, since everyone responds so differently."

Then, the flurry of activity returned as Adam coded. He was dying. The nurses rushed him down to the operating room once more, and Julie and her family anxiously waited, unprepared for what would come next. "We got the most horrible news," said Julie. "The doctors told us that because of the lack of blood flow, and Adam's infection, they had no choice but to amputate both of his legs above the ankles, and his left hand. We were just sick to our stomachs."

Julie said that during the first fifteen days that they were at Walter Reed, Adam coded seven times. His liver failed, his kidneys failed, and he was placed on dialysis.

Though the doctors were experienced in traumatic war wounds and were doing all they could to save Adam, they told Julie and her family they should prepare to say good-bye to him. Things just kept getting progressively worse. "The chaplain was coming in all of the time, and there were lots of social workers. It was terrible! I remember being in the waiting room and having a conversation with a brother of a soldier who was also in the hospital like Adam. As we were consoling each other, we heard 'code blue' on the loud speaker. We instinctively both jumped up and ran to the nurse's station, where they told us it was another wounded warrior. You just react," Julie said.

Julie had the feeling that the doctors had all but given up hope. "None of them could look me in the eye," said Julie. "I had nurses patting me on my shoulder all of the time, and everyone had such sad looks on their faces. I was furious! 'He's not dead,' I told them. I said to the doctors that if they didn't come into Adam's room with hope in their eyes, then I don't want them there at all!

"I am not one for confrontation, but you change when it is your child. I actually said to one doctor: 'Get out of here; I can't deal with your sad face.' "

Fortunately, Julie had the unrelenting support of Stephen, who was with her full-time, and who also looked after their house, and took care of all of the details that Julie just couldn't handle. Her nephew, Daniel, who was like a brother to Adam, left his job, taking all the vacation days he could to be by Adam's side. His sister came to the hospital immediately from California on July 15 and stayed with the family through December. The love and devotion of her family was paramount for Julie's physical and mental well-being and Adam's long and trying recovery.

Following the amputations, and because of his skin condition, the doctors decided to transfer Adam to the University of Maryland Medical Center's Shock Trauma Unit. As they prepared to move him by helicopter,

Adam coded again in his bed. They stabilized him and radioed for another helicopter—this one with a larger respirator. As they prepared to move him a second time, Adam coded once more. Finally, they were able to keep him stable and begin the short ride to Baltimore. When Adam arrived, he was in such bad shape that they couldn't take him to the operating room right away as they had hoped.

Adam, thankfully, stabilized overnight, and the next day went into surgery to remove the massive amount of dead skin from his body. "They were able to do only the left side during this surgery, as it is a very long and painful procedure," said Julie. The family met with Dr. Sharon Henry after surgery, and because of Adam's extremely weak condition, the extensive surgeries that lay ahead, and his severe brain injury, they were told he may or may not recover. "No one really knew how to proceed from this point, and all we could do was wait and see how he did over the weekend," said Julie.

Adam remained stable, so on Monday the surgeons, including Dr. Joseph Dubois, went in and operated on his right side. From then he was in surgery three days a week for wound dressing changes and, subsequently, skin grafts. During one procedure they went in to clean the wounds on his right leg and discovered that the bone had partially died. They would have to revise the amputation.

"I guess if there was any silver lining, it was that the doctors told us Adam had some viable skin on the dead leg, and that they could use that skin for more grafts on other parts of his body. He had lost so much skin they didn't know where they would get all the grafts he needed. Even with this, they had to stretch all of the new skin over his wounds as far as they could for maximal coverage. They did amazing work on him, and, eventually, he was able to be taken off of dialysis and his respirator, and they could finally insert a tracheostomy. Lucky for us, there was an unexpected tiny air pocket in the tube, so it allowed Adam to speak to us for the very first time. He said: 'Where am I?' Everyone just went crazy!"

As any parent or loved one of someone who has suffered a TBI knows, predicting what his or her personality will be like after the injury is difficult at best. "They told us that there would be a possibility that he would not be who he was before," Julie said. "But we knew he was there." Julie searched the Internet for everything she could find on brain injuries. "I realized that there would be the possibility that he wouldn't be the same, but I really felt that he was going to be okay." And, luckily, he was.

With Julie by his side, Adam began to significantly improve during the five months he spent in Baltimore. The Army would come to visit Adam every couple of weeks to monitor his progress, and there was much to be hopeful about in his prognosis and recovery. Adam returned to Walter Reed for rehabilitation. In August 2011, he was transferred to San Antonio, Texas, for two months for specialized wound care. "It was kind of funny, but we missed being at Walter Reed because we had so many friends there, and the guys who were being treated had suffered as a result of the War on Terror. We actually were very much looking forward to getting back," Julie said.

A few weeks later, Adam returned to Walter Reed, and Julie was happy to be reunited with her Mighty Mom friends and all of the organizations that helped them since they first arrived.

"The Aleethia Foundation is another organization that we love. They take the wounded warriors and their caregivers out for Friday night dinners," said Julie. These would become events that both the moms and their sons and daughters would eagerly anticipate.

"We were so excited to go to our first Friday night dinner," said Julie. She was happy to finally get a break and take a much-needed respite from the hospital. "We had been in the hospital for over ten months, and we were really looking forward to it. We got Adam all ready, and finally made it onto the bus," Julie said. As the group left for dinner, the bus hit a large bump in the road, and Adam felt excruciating pain from the impact. "I thought to myself, 'Oh no, this is not good,' but we still managed to make it to the restaurant."

When wounded warriors take trips outside of the hospital, the Navy makes sure there is always a nurse with the group, and Julie mentioned to her that Adam was really hurting. The nurse checked him to see if she could help him with anything, and Julie decided to give Adam some painkillers. While Julie knew that he would be fine through dinner, she was more than concerned about the return trip. "I was very worried about Adam taking the bus back, but the Aleethia Foundation said not to worry. They ordered a cab to pick us up that was wheelchair accessible and would be easier considering Adam's fragile state at the time. This was the first time I ever talked to Aleethia, and they were just great. They not only arranged for the cab, but paid for it too," Julie said. "We have attended many of these dinners since, and everyone at the foundation has become just like family."

Another nonprofit, the Yellow Ribbon Fund, where Julie eventually started working part-time, among other things, organizes special caregiver dinners. The moms especially appreciated these get-togethers. "The Yellow Ribbon Fund does it all—arranges the meals, provides transportation, and takes care of any other particular needs of the family," Julie added.

The good news was that Adam was continuing to heal. The bad news was that his marriage was, sadly, falling apart.

"Rosie, Courtney, and I had flown to Walter Reed together on July 20, 2010. Rosie stayed with Adam for just over five months. She went home several times, including on Thanksgiving and Christmas, but returned to spend New Year's Eve with him. Adam was transferred back to Walter Reed on January 5, 2011, and Rosie traveled with him in the ambulance. She stayed until January 9, left to go home, and said she would be back next weekend, but she didn't come," Julie said.

In the beginning of February, Rosie did come back one last time to visit Adam.

"I was in the room, as usual, and thought maybe I should go out for a few hours to give them some time alone," said Julie. "So I told Adam that I would be back in a couple of hours, and to call if he needed me. Halfway down the hall I realized that I had forgotten something and went back to his room to pick it up. When I walked in, Adam was crying hysterically, and I screamed, 'What is going on?' And she goes, 'We are just talking,' and I looked at Adam and said, 'Do you need me to stay?' He goes, 'I'll be fine, Mom.' So I left and I kept thinking that she is his wife, and if he wants to work it out with her, well, that's okay because he must need her. When I came back from my errands I asked her where she was going, because I saw her put on her coat. She replied, 'Home.' "

That was the last time Julie and Adam saw Rosie. Then in May 2011, Adam got a text message from Rosie. It simply said: "Just send me the divorce papers!" Adam and Rosie's marriage was over, and they were eventually legally divorced.

After fifteen months as an inpatient, on November 5, Adam and Julie got the good news that he was going to be discharged. Adam would move into Building 62, where wounded warriors who are outpatients live during rehabilitation. "Everyone was so happy, and the doctors and nurses were clapping and cheering because they were so thrilled for Adam," said Julie.

"We finally left the hospital and were heading through the garage to get to the apartment, when Adam had a seizure. We called for an ambulance, went to the emergency room, and then there we were—back in his room on the fourth floor of the hospital. They hadn't even taken his name off the door, and we were back," Julie said. This was the third of five seizures that Adam would suffer, adding to the anxiety that the family would feel, and the roller-coaster recovery process that Adam endured since his injury.

But Adam had an incredible ability to withstand great pain, fear, loss, and uncertainty, thanks to the grace he inherited from his mom, as well as his overall good nature. "It's so hard to explain why Adam has such a positive attitude," said Julie. "He's always been positive and upbeat and loves what he is doing, so there is no blame there. He knew at some point he could get hurt. Like all of the other moms here, we knew that at some level, too, but we just don't think about it. If you do, it will drive you crazy."

Even as an outpatient, Adam had injuries that were very complex and difficult to treat, and the healing process was slow and full of unexpected hurdles. His belly was open, covered only with mesh and skin grafts. He developed a large hernia and had to wear a hernia belt, which was not good for his comfort or self-esteem. If the doctors continued on the same path, Adam would just have basic skin grafts, but his skin would be very fragile, and one unexpected incident could send him right back to the hospital. The doctors were trying desperately to develop a new game plan. Then, in March 2013, Adam was admitted back into the hospital to have his abdomen closed. Unfortunately, the preliminary procedure failed, his liver was damaged, and he ended up in the ICU.

Finally, the doctors came up with an idea to completely close Adam's abdomen, but the procedure could be life-threatening. "Adam and I talked and talked and talked, and he said that he really wanted the operation, despite the possibility of so many unknowns. I was so nervous," said Julie.

Adam went in for surgery again on October 28, 2013. Dr. Carlos Rodriguez, his general surgeon, had met with Dr. Lee Valerio from plastic surgery. Together, with their respective teams, they decided to use a new procedure. "Everything went better than anticipated, and they were able to pull the muscles together in one eleven-hour surgery. Adam would, however, still need a skin graft on this wound," Julie added.

Dr. Valerio wanted to try something called Spray-On Skin, a procedure that had only been used on burn victims, and was not FDA-approved for trauma patients such as Adam. It is used for wounds that don't heal after three months. Doctors take skin cells from the patient, mix them in a patented solution, and then spray it on the affected area. "I told Dr. Valerio that we would love to be the test case for using the Spray-On Skin on Adam, and that if it could help other wounded warriors, I would be thrilled," Julie said.

Initially, it was unclear if the procedure could be used. But waiting was not an option for this Mighty Mom. "As luck would have it, I heard that Adam was going to have a visit from President Barack Obama in just a few days. I thought, 'This is my chance.'"

As with any presidential visit, the advance team arrives first. "One member of President Obama's advance team came in the room and told us what to expect and asked if they could do anything for us. I said, 'Actually, there is something you can do for us,' and I proceeded to tell her about the spray skin and how much we wanted to use it on Adam, but that it wasn't FDA-approved for non-burn patients. She was very nice and said that I could certainly bring it up with the president, but that she would most likely be the person following up," said Julie. The president's aide suggested that Julie send her an email and handed her a business card.

Later that day, President Obama met with Adam, and right before he was ready to leave, he asked Julie if there was anything he could do for them. "I said: 'Thank you, Mr. President. I did speak to your assistant and will be sending her an email about a procedure.'" That Monday, Julie got a response from the aide, and she said they would be looking into it. One week later, Dr. Valerio happily informed Adam and Julie that he was given approval to use the Spray-On Skin on a one-time basis only. "It doesn't matter who you approach or how nervous you are when you are doing it for your child," Julie said.

"The thing is, I knew this was going to work because Adam is feeling good, his blood work was fine, and he was eating. This was a good sign. Finally, we will have a surgery that will be going as planned," said Julie. "You know Adam had nearly 140 surgeries up to this point, and I was so hopeful that this one might be his last."

In November 2103, Adam's experimental procedure took place. It was very successful, according to Julie, but the doctors still had to wait a full week to see if the skin was beginning to grow and if the wound had covered. "We were on pins and needles," said Julie, "but we were very optimistic. Adam looked great."

As Dr. Valerio removed the dressing, everyone in the room was silent. Julie hoped that the procedure worked and that Adam would be able to get on with his rehabilitation process and start getting back to a more normal life. As the doctor took the first peek at Adam, everyone could see the broad smile on his face. He said everything looked "great." The procedure was a success! For Julie, it was a miracle. She was ecstatic. Adam was beginning the next chapter on the road to his recovery. Julie was relieved and thrilled for Adam. Her son—who soldiered on through countless surgeries, near-death experiences, excruciating pain, and emotional distress—was now in a good place.

Mothers are a rare breed. Mothers of wounded warriors, however, are a national treasure.

"I think all of the moms who are here with their wounded warriors are very special people," Julie said. "I get that if you are a wife or a girlfriend that they might not be able to handle this, but a mother has no option, as far as I am concerned," Julie said. "I don't think mothers have an alternative; it is your child!"

Julie said that the Mighty Moms gravitate to each other because they, tragically, share a common bond. "We need to have someone to understand what we are going through, and it doesn't matter what injury their kids have. We are going through the same things, living together in the same building, and even though we talk to the wives here, only another mother knows what you are going through.

"Sometimes we all end up laughing, or we can all end up crying, which is good for us," Julie continued. "But you know when you are talking to that person they get it. I am lucky to have a sister who is my best friend, and another very close girlfriend who was always there for me. Even though I can call them at two in the morning—and, believe me, when you are here you have no sense of time—they can't 100 percent relate. But the moms here live this every day, and they can see by the look on your face what you are feeling and what you are going through."

Sharing is the common denominator among the Mighty Moms of Walter Reed. Whether it is providing information, giving social advice, or baking apple pies, these moms help not only their wounded warriors, but each other, too.

"It's all about sharing," Julie said. "It's like the thing with the spray skin with Adam. It opens the door for the next person who may need this kind of skin graft. So, yes, in the scheme of things, it is for everybody. We sometimes will sit around and say, 'This happened to my son,' and someone will say, 'Well, this is what happened with my son.' We exchange information on medical procedures, and what has helped our child. We need to help each other, and when a new mom comes here, we try to tell them everything they need to know."

Julie said that one of the observations she has made over the years is that people group the wounded warriors by their respective injuries. "They tend to refer to our kids as double amps, or triple amps, and that gets us crazy," Julie said. Each of these wounded warriors is a unique individual with unique and individual injuries. "The mothers turn into crazy people when they are fighting for their children. The great thing about being a mom and not a wife is that we don't have to worry about our children's careers, so we just don't care. For us it doesn't matter how many medals you have on your chest. If I need to say something to you, I am going to say it. They may not always like us, but I hope they realize that when you are a mom that protective instinct kicks in almost automatically. The military doesn't intimidate us," Julie added.

The Mighty Moms fiercely advocate for their children. They routinely attend Town Hall and caregiver meetings and are vocal about what they believe is working and what needs to change. After all, many are professionals themselves—Siobhan McConnell is an attorney, Tammy Karcher a document specialist, and Julie a lab technician, and the others have a wealth of experience that they put to work on behalf of their injured sons and daughters. "I have seen mothers in Town Hall meetings get up and ask questions exactly the right way, but if they don't get the response they want, they completely change," Julie said, knowing the inner beast firsthand. "The thing is that we don't hide anything. If we see something that needs to be changed, we follow the chain of command, but if we need to, we will go over their heads."

"We have become quite a good team, and even though we are from all walks of life, we have grown together like family," Julie said. "We see each other all of the time, and when we go to events we are always together. While we don't always hang out at each other's apartments, we know we can call each other anytime. The truth is that some moms you get really close to, but regardless, there is nothing we wouldn't do to help each other."

The Mighty Moms have their own chain of command too, but at any one time, a mom could be the general or a private first class. The group is egalitarian, and their main mission is to inform, protect, and love. "When we meet new moms for the first time, they have no idea that they can fly their loved ones here for free or get financial assistance," Julie said. "So we talk to them and give them advice on what services are available and all the support that people so generously provide to the families of wounded warriors. You need that support, especially when they are here all alone."

"Sometimes when I think about our group I just have to laugh, since we are all so very different. Ramona Wasylenko and I probably would never have been friends." Ramona's son, Mark, is a wounded warrior who was also treated at Walter Reed and is now medically retired. "She is from Boston, and let's just say she is very assertive—but I love her. She made me laugh, and we cried so many times together, or sometimes we made complete fools out of ourselves. She would never judge me. Now that she is back home, she has friends, but no one can understand her like us. And Stacy works on a farm. I have never even been on a farm. But I know I can call Stacy anytime and she will be there for me. I learned to never judge a book by its cover," Julie said.

While it seems ridiculous to try to find any good that has come out of being catastrophically injured in war, Julie, like all of the Mighty Moms, hangs onto the belief that there is much good that can come from tragedy.

For Julie, there have been many blessings, foremost being that Adam is alive. "To have Adam with us, given what he has been through, is a miracle," Julie said. "I always have to look at the good part of this entire situation. Adam and I have always been close, but now we can sit in a room and look at each other and know what the other one needs without saying a word. We always did things together as a family, but now it means even more," Julie said.

"One time he said to me, 'Mom, I'm worried that you and Dad have spent so much time away from each other because of me.' I told him, 'Honey, Dad and I have been married for thirty-two years, and you don't have to worry.' "

Julie knows that while Adam still needs her for many things, he is also a twenty-nine-year-old man who needs his independence. "One day when he was going to rehab, we were ready to leave the apartment and he turned to me and said he could do this by himself. So I took off my coat and sat down. Then I went outside and watched him go, then went back into the apartment and had a good cry."

Julie said that another high point of Adam's experience is her access to a president, a first lady, and a host of famous people. "Hey, I got to go to the

Inaugural Ball," Julie said. "That would never happen to me in my normal life. We've met so many people like movie stars and sports figures. I would never have had the opportunity to go to so many sports events, and also to meet so many wonderful nonprofit organizations. I would never have done that."

Julie said that she hopes the American people can look at Adam and be comfortable talking to him. "Some people stare at Adam, and I know he may look a little odd. But, he is very comfortable in his own skin, and accepts his new life quite happily. My hope is that people, when they see him, will come over and thank him for his service. He enjoys talking to people and doesn't want anyone to feel sorry for him. Just don't stare at him or look away," Julie added.

But Adam's sense of humor is boundless. He had T-shirts made with these phrases on the front: I DID IT FOR THE PARKING; TAKE A PICTURE, IT LASTS LONGER; or SHARK ATTACK. Adam uses his humor to engage with other people. Julie said she thinks Adam, who has done a good amount of public speaking, would be a "terrific motivator."

"Adam is a compelling speaker, and he wants to become a peer mentor and help other wounded warriors adjust to their new lives," said Julie. "He purchased some land in Annapolis, Maryland, and he will have a new house built there so he can be close to his doctors and also live in a military-friendly environment."

For Julie, her dream is to simply get back to a normal life. "My husband teases me that there will be no red carpet when I get back home," Julie said as she sipped her cup of coffee. "This is what I look most forward to. I want to go back and live with my husband, get up on a Sunday morning with no makeup on, and drink a cup of coffee. Then, I want to do the *New York Times* crossword puzzle and keep my bathrobe on all day."

NINE

STEFANIE D. MASON AND PAULETTE MASON

I F ANYONE HAD REASON TO BELIEVE SHE UNDERSTOOD THE MILITARY, AND could use that knowledge in an emergency, it was Paulette Mason. After all, her call to duty came not long after her daughter Stefanie joined the Army Reserve. Unfortunately, being familiar with the military wasn't enough after Stefanie was badly injured in Afghanistan. There were as many surprises in the recovery process as there were on day one, when Paulette first learned of her daughter's enlistment.

"Stefanie came home one day and announced she'd be leaving to go into the Army," said Paulette, who lives with her husband in Newark, Delaware. "She informed us that she had just joined the Army Reserve, and my husband and I went, 'You did what?' This was just after the war in Iraq had started, and she said, 'Don't worry. The war's going to be over.' I said, 'I am worried,' and I think I started crying after that."

To the family's surprise, Stefanie had already completed her in-processing paperwork in Baltimore. The next step was basic training at Fort Jackson, in South Carolina, and advanced individual training to become a logistical specialist at Fort Lee in Virginia.

"I was angry and remember that I couldn't even talk to her about what she had done," Paulette said. "Finally, after a few days, I calmed down and accepted the fact that this was her life, and it was what she wanted to do." But there were still questions. "I thought, what's the Army Reserve?" Paulette said. "I knew nothing about the military."

She soon had plenty of opportunities to learn.

Once Stefanie was assigned to the 485th Chemical Battalion in Wilmington, Delaware, she volunteered her mom for the unit's "Family Readiness Group." The idea was to have family members help each other as they learned the ways of the Army Reserve while the troops were at home and, even more importantly, to be there for each other should the 485th be deployed to one of the two active hot spots at the time, Iraq and Afghanistan. Paulette, a vice president of marketing and public relations for a local accounting firm, was put in charge of the group's newsletter.

"It was a very loose group," Paulette said. "Because there was no deployment, there wasn't really much going on for us to get involved."

That didn't last long. Stefanie received notice that she would be heading for Iraq, but not with her chemical battalion. She was being assigned to a Wheeling, West Virginia, unit, the 463rd Combat Engineer Battalion. They deployed to Balad Air Base in October 2004. The base, which at one time during the war was home to about twenty-eight thousand troops, would become the largest logistical support center for coalition forces in Iraq. It was located forty miles north of Baghdad, in the heart of the Sunni Triangle, where the insurgency was in full swing when Stefanie arrived. Contrary to the hopes of many just the year before, it was now clear the war would not end quickly. Though Paulette had been preparing to help keep families informed when it was the 485th's turn to be shipped overseas, there wasn't much information sharing when Stefanie was sent to another battalion.

"There was very little communication from the group, but I tried to keep up," Paulette said. "I can't tell much about the deployment other than I was so stressed because it was a bad time over there."

But Paulette isn't the type of person to sit at home and fret. She found an outlet for her worries.

"I was a mess, so I decided to take karate," Paulette said. And she's used to the look of disbelief from people when she tells the story. "You're laughing. I know. People looked at me. I was a tennis player. But the only way to handle the stress was to start beating up on that bag. And sparring was the only way to calm me down. So I sparred my way to a black belt in four years." Even better, a proud Stefanie would be there when her mother passed the black belt test.

After fifteen months in Iraq, Stefanie was back in Delaware, both as a reservist with the 485th, and as a civilian court employee working for the state. Paulette's stress level was down considerably, thanks to karate, and oft-repeated reassurances from the Department of Defense that National Guard and Reserve units should expect to see only one deployment every five years. Unfortunately, though Stefanie had recently completed one deployment, her Wilmington chemical battalion had not, and it was alerted in 2007 that it would be heading for Kuwait.

In the meantime, Paulette had taken on additional duties with the military, volunteering to be the Delaware publicity chair for a Defense Department program called the Employer Support of the Guard and Reserve (ESGR), a nationwide network of volunteers that works with guard members and reservists and their employers to sort through problems that arise as a result of an employee's military responsibilities. "I wanted to learn as much as possible," Paulette said, "and the Department of Defense program was another way for me to become more informed on Reserve issues and the military."

During Stefanie's second deployment, Paulette volunteered once again for "mom duty" with the 485th, this time as leader of the Family Readiness Group. Unlike the first stint, when she was urged on by her daughter, this move was inspired in part by what Paulette saw all too often as a military mom. "I never thought the military communicated very well to families," Paulette said. "And being a writer and communicator, I had a pretty good idea of how to do it right."

Though at this point communications was a natural role for her, it was actually Paulette's second career. Her first degree, in bioscience, from Delaware Technical Community College, led to a career in pharmaceutical research at AstraZeneca. Seeking a career change after her divorce, she earned a communications degree from the University of Delaware. Though Paulette considered doing some graduate work, she was in her mid-thirties and had five-year-old twin girls to support—Stefanie and her sister, Jennifer. Paulette went to work for DuPont, first writing chemistry instrumentation manuals for chemical analyzers, and then moving to a marketing communications position for DuPont Merck Pharmaceuticals.

"It was very difficult going back to college, because I was thirty-five years old, a single mom, holding a part-time job, and raising twin daughters," Paulette said. "But I graduated and was even named the outstanding department of communications graduating senior. It was a bittersweet moment. They wanted me to do graduate work, but I couldn't because I had two kids to support and raise."

After leaving DuPont, she worked for a time for the Wilmington *News Journal* and did freelance work before landing another full-time marketing position.

"I was hired by a local accounting firm," Paulette said. "With my background from industry, I had a pretty good idea of how to do trade shows and how to write. I did brochures, layout and design, sales development, and marketing. I did that for eight years, and then one of the partners left and started his own firm, and I became vice president of marketing for him. That was for ten years. I loved doing that. He was a great guy to work for. My new position further enhanced my business skills and helped me focus on building my leadership and networking skills. It also gave me the opportunity to volunteer in the community. And my volunteering was with the military and Department of Defense."

It was her initial volunteering with Stefanie's unit, and the interaction it brought with state officials and US senators, as well as her work with ESGR, that led to her appointment to chair Delaware's ESGR efforts and join the group's national committee on strategic planning. It was work she enjoyed, and continued, even after Stefanie's tour of duty in Kuwait ended in 2008.

By the time of Stefanie's third call-up in 2009, Paulette was very involved in ESGR. She acted as liaison between employers and the military and kept both up to date on shared concerns. She organized information sessions and seminars for employers, coordinated trips to local bases to familiarize them with the work of the troops, or sent reminders that the law protected the jobs of returning members of the Guard and Reserve. It was a long way from writing newsletters and doing publicity.

"I started out at the grassroots, being a mom doing this or that, but this was a protocol position of a two-star general," Paulette said. "So instead of being in the audience, all of a sudden I became chair of a state organization, and when I was going to a function, I was sitting with the two-star or the senators. All of a sudden I was in their company or doing presentations to them on the state of ESGR affairs in Delaware for the Guard and Reserve."

The assignment made sense professionally, allowing her to put her marketing skills to work for the troops. "I would always look at something and say, 'How could we improve it? Could we do better?' As a professional, and working with the military, I could see that they had problems with communications, always have."

She's proud of her team's outreach to the state's business community. "My job was to engage the employers in a positive manner so that we could cut down on problems of having soldiers fired," Paulette said. "I think we really built the program up in Delaware. We would actually invite employers to a day in the life of the troops. We took employers up on an airplane, a C-5 cargo aircraft. I worked closely with the command of the Delaware National Guard and Dover Air Force Base and had many resources at my disposal."

Then, six years into her eight-year Reserve commitment, Stefanie received an alert for deployment number three: Afghanistan. "And that was where everything started," Paulette said.

First, this mom was not too happy about another overseas assignment for her daughter. And now, with years of experience dealing with the military, from the unit level to general officers and civilian officials at the Pentagon, she felt more than comfortable speaking her mind. "This was three deployments in six years—right—after—another," Paulette said, emphasizing the last three words by pounding the table—one pound for each word. In her work with ESGR, she was regularly traveling to Washington, and she often heard the undersecretary of defense for Reserve Affairs talk about the policy of one deployment every five years. At one meeting, she raised her hand and asked him to explain what that meant. When he did, she fired back, "Well, why is my daughter now going on her third deployment?" As she recalls, "He didn't respond, and everybody looked at me, but I didn't care."

The third deployment arose, in part, as a result of Stefanie seeking a different assignment. After Kuwait, she wanted to work in civil affairs—the branch of the military that acts in a war zone as a liaison between the troops and the local civilian population—and she was reassigned to the 352nd Civil Affairs Command based in Fort Meade, Maryland. Not long after, in September 2009, word came that she would be assigned to another unit, the 354th Civil Affairs Command, which was preparing to deploy to Afghanistan. In two weeks, she was to report to Fort Dix, New Jersey. That was October 4, the same day as the Army Ten-Miler, an annual run held in Washington, DC, that she had been training for all summer. Stefanie, a standout athlete, had missed the Ten-Miler in previous years because of other deployments, and she had hoped to dedicate that year's run to Sergeant Joseph Nurre, a fellow soldier who had been killed during her deployment to Iraq. She expressed her disappointment to her mom—the mom who was already unhappy about a third overseas tour, and who had a black belt in karate, and who was no longer the least bit shy about expressing concerns to top brass.

"Stefanie and I were at a function in Washington," Paulette said, "and I went right up to the general in charge of the Army Reserves at that time and said, 'General, my daughter just got two weeks' notice, and she wants to run in the Army Ten-Miler, but they said she had to leave that day.' And then we went to another secretary. It came back that they let her run, and she reported to Fort Dix that evening. But she got to run, and she did well. She was in the top 10 percent. She's a great runner."

The 354th arrived for duty as part of the International Joint Command headquarters in Kabul, Afghanistan, in January 2010, and Stefanie was enjoying working with military representatives from NATO countries and other allies. "It was the greatest experience," she would later say. "I loved it, and I thought, 'This is where I belong.'"

Four months after their arrival, on April 20, Staff Sergeant Stefanie Mason was riding in an up-armor SUV, in the front passenger seat, when the driver lost control of the vehicle and it crashed head on into a concrete wall. Stefanie's seatbelt didn't work, and she smashed headfirst into the thick, bulletproof windshield. She suffered a traumatic brain injury, nine facial fractures including a broken jaw, a tibia plateau fracture (where her leg crashed into the dashboard), and a degenerated disc in her back. "I had two hematomas on the brain, and it was swelling so much they were going to cut my skull open to relieve the pressure," Stefanie said. "But when they put me in an induced coma, the brain stopped swelling. I have to thank the French doctors at the base for saving my life. They were the ones responsible for me right after the accident."

Paulette got the dreaded call that evening.

"I just remember my husband and I were sitting in the family room," Paulette recalled. "And at ten thirty at night, the phone call came in and we saw the telephone number flash up on the television screen, and I thought, 'That's weird. That's coming from one of the Air Force bases.'" She assumed it was ESGR business and picked up. She didn't recognize the officer who identified himself, and she asked what unit he was from.

"I'm from your daughter's civil affairs unit in Afghanistan," Paulette remembered hearing. "I wanted to let you know that your daughter was in an accident, and she's been a bit banged up."

"Is she alive?"

"Yes, she's a bit banged up, but I don't know her condition."

Paulette wanted to speak to someone who could be more specific, and the officer promised to have someone call. Two hours later—seemingly a lifetime—the phone rang again. Despite her overall state of shock, Paulette said she was able to follow the neurosurgeon's report, in part thanks to her medical writing background. He told her there had been an accident, that Stefanie's head had hit the windshield. She had a brain injury, and was in critical condition at Bagram Air Base, where she had been moved from Kabul. "We're going to have to wait and see," he said.

"Is she going to make it through the night?" Paulette wanted to know.

"We're going to have to wait and see," he repeated. "That's all I can tell you."

Paulette said, "I remember crying, and then just picking up my rosary and going to bed, and just praying myself to sleep. That's what I did. I prayed myself to sleep, asking the Blessed Mother not to take my daughter.

"I'm still numb from the whole thing," she said more than three years later. "I know my husband just held me and said, 'That's all we can do. We have to wait until morning.' "

She did, but not a second longer. She made a number of calls, including to the head of the National Guard in Delaware. Then she called ESGR's office in Washington. "Stefanie has been injured, but I don't know what's going on," she told them. ESGR immediately contacted a public relations specialist who had worked for them but was now in Bagram and asked if she could look for Stefanie. A few hours later, the woman, Beth, called Paulette. "I'm sitting here at Stefanie's bedside," she said. "I'm holding her hand. She doesn't know what's going on, and she's in and out of consciousness. But she wants to talk to you." The next thing Paulette knew, Stefanie was on the phone saying, "Mom, I need you."

"That's all she said to me, and it just broke my heart," Paulette said. "I couldn't do anything. I felt helpless, even with all these great connections."

One connection, at least, had made a difference. "I knew Beth was there at her bedside, giving Stefanie comfort. And Beth was saying, 'I know your mom, I work with your mom.' And she was holding Stefanie's hand. She said it just put Stefanie at peace, and that's . . . I don't know if Stefanie remembers that. She doesn't remember much from that at all, but she remembers somebody being there."

Aside from the call from Stefanie's unit, the family still hadn't heard from the Army Reserve. And there were still so many questions to answer.

What was Stefanie's condition? Where would they send her? When? What should the family do? But other calls were coming in, from the governor's office and from Delaware's US senators. Just the week before, US Senator Tom Carper, of Delaware, who was in Afghanistan, had visited Stefanie. Paulette has the picture of her daughter giving Carper a big hug. "I had everybody calling me that day," Paulette said. "Everybody knew that Stefanie was hurt, but I still hadn't heard from the Army Reserve."

Finally, on day two, casualty affairs called. "When is she coming home?" Paulette wanted to know. Stefanie wasn't stable enough to travel. And there was another complication: a gigantic ash cloud resulting from the eruption of an Icelandic volcano the week before had disrupted air travel throughout Europe. Tens of thousands of flights were canceled, stranding millions of travelers. It wasn't immediately clear if Stefanie could be moved to the Landstuhl hospital in Germany, or if she would have to go elsewhere. But even from a distance, Paulette was working with the doctors on making decisions about her daughter's treatment. In one case, she insisted that they wait to operate on Stefanie's leg until she reached the States. There were many more calls about possible arrival dates before Stefanie finally made it to Walter Reed late one evening. Paulette was by her side the next day.

"Her sister came down with me," Paulette said. "And Jennifer and I made our way to Walter Reed hospital. We found out she was in the ICU, and Jennifer just had her arms around me to hold me up because we didn't know what we were going to see."

They saw tubes, lots of them, and a battered and bruised Stefanie.

Paulette said, "Her leg was just totally bandaged, and in a straight cast. But her face was so messed up. It was so swollen. She had two raccoon eyes. She just looked horrible, and she couldn't talk because her jaw was broken. She couldn't eat. She couldn't move her lips. And she could hardly see because everything was spinning and she had double vision. She wouldn't even open her eyes sometimes because she was so sick to her stomach.

"I went into mom mode, saying, 'What can I do?' " Paulette said. "I didn't cry or anything like that. I started asking questions about her medical condition."

Those next few days, in the intensive care unit and later when Stefanie was moved to a room, were a blur for Paulette. She remembers a stream of well-wishers, from her daughter's unit at nearby Fort Meade and others, but Paulette can't remember whom she met or to whom she spoke. She does remember finally asking for some privacy. "It was too much," Paulette said.

"At this point, I just needed to focus on my daughter." She would do that, in person, for a few days, and then head home to catch up with work. Then it was back to Walter Reed. She was in Delaware when she learned from her daughter that she was being transferred to the Hunter Holmes McGuire VA Medical Center in Richmond, Virginia. "I knew Stefanie had a head injury, but I didn't know how bad it was," Paulette said. "McGuire is big for spinal cord and head trauma, and she was being sent there for intense therapy for her traumatic brain injury, for the cognition problems, for the seeing problems, the balance. She couldn't walk because of her leg, but she was also dizzy all the time. So they were trying to do some things with the brain."

The problem was that the people in charge didn't alert Paulette, who had been expecting to join her daughter at Walter Reed again for a few days. Paulette was being painfully reminded of all the communications issues she'd encountered during her volunteer days with the Reserves.

"They forgot to tell us," Paulette said. "I didn't know what was going on. I didn't even know what to ask. So the next thing we know she's in Richmond, and we're traveling four hours down Interstate 95 every weekend because she's in a hospital down there and they wouldn't let me stay with her."

When the Army did become more communicative, Paulette was floored by the news. When Stefanie returned to Walter Reed after a couple of months in Richmond, Paulette would need to be with her daughter full-time, as a nonmedical attendant. She was told to report to the Mologne House, a short-term lodging facility on the hospital grounds, at 2:00 p.m. on June 30. That was when Stefanie was due in from Richmond, and they could check in together then.

"I didn't know what to say," Paulette said.

She was there—on time. However, the military did not show up with Stefanie until three hours later.

"I should've known from that day that they never did anything on time," Paulette said.

June 30 marked the start of Paulette and Stefanie living together again full-time for the next three years.

"June 30 she came to live at the Mologne House, and we stayed until August 2011," Paulette said. "Then we moved to Bethesda, when they closed down the old Walter Reed, and into Building 62. We left in January of 2013, so she was in outpatient therapy since June 30, 2010. All this, as that colonel said, because she was 'a bit banged up.' I would say so."

Over time, Paulette learned to ask questions, to speak up for her daughter, and to not take anything for granted. It was a different Paulette who, reflecting on her daughter's experiences, later jotted down notes about the time after Stefanie was hurt. Of that first day at the Mologne House, she wrote:

> "No more weekend trips to Richmond. No more crying because I had to leave her behind. . . . What a way for a mother to live. . . . Finally we will be together so I can take care of her and tell her how much I love her.
>
> No one is talking to me. I'm just staring at everything. There are a lot of people that come and go, but no one ever says hi and I'm afraid to ask anything.
>
> Finally, I see my daughter. She's being wheeled in her wheelchair by a guy in a military uniform. I go to greet her. She looks terrible. Her two black eyes are still puffy and her mouth is still drooping on one side. I'm still not over the shock of her injuries. Yet with all that is going on, and how she appears, she still manages to say, 'I love you, Mom. Thanks for being here.' "

Living in a small room with two double beds would prove to be an adventure for Paulette. Stefanie was in a wheelchair for at least eight months. If she wanted to maneuver herself into bed or the shower, her mom would carry the injured leg while Stefanie hopped about on the other one. Paulette thought the rooms were dirty, wet, and moldy—she would insist on three moves in their eighteen months there. Yet she has high praise for the civilian staff. "Wonderful," she called them. "They cared. They really did care."

She would not always feel that way about the military, and its rules and expectations for her injured daughter. Paulette's priority was to help Stefanie recover, not to ensure that she followed protocol. And while her staff sergeant daughter couldn't talk back, her mom sure could.

"My daughter had a traumatic brain injury, and with a brain injury you sleep a lot," Paulette said. "You can't stay awake, and your hours are irregular, and she's in pain with her leg. And they're talking about an eight o'clock formation. I said, 'Are you crazy?' They wanted all the soldiers in formation, and I said, 'My daughter is not going to formation. She goes to bed sometimes at three o'clock in the morning. She's on morphine. You're not having her sign papers, and she's not going to formation. I will go, but she will not.'

"So that's how I got to be as mean as I am. That was my child. When she went into the military, she was in perfect shape. When she came home, she was like this. I was looking out for her welfare."

The medical side raised concerns for her as well. Though Paulette had been drafted to be Stefanie's nonmedical attendant, she never felt adequately briefed on what would be required of her once they moved into the Mologne House. She was never informed about an orientation for her new assignment or kept up to date on what would come next. She never saw anything remotely resembling a care plan, which the hospital promises patients on its website.

"I didn't know she had appointments, or how the appointments were set up," Paulette said. "Those in charge were setting up follow-up appointments, which she couldn't remember, and they didn't tell me. So we missed them. There were no calls or reminders."

As this was the military, missing an appointment was akin to not reporting for scheduled duty, and Stefanie was threatened with an Article 15, a nonjudicial punishment similar to a misdemeanor in civilian courts. "I said, 'Wait a minute, what are you guys doing here?' " Paulette said. "I start getting the drift real fast that they are totally disorganized. . . . I don't know how they win wars. I really don't."

She found Walter Reed "survival guides" on the Internet and studied those and started doing her own research on Stefanie's wounds and treatment. She insisted on a printout of Stefanie's medications. She wanted to schedule appointments—for physical therapy, for occupational therapy, for the dentist and eye doctor, and for neuropsychology—around what worked for Stefanie. "I said, 'How about I make them, and I can put her on a schedule because she sleeps a lot?' I was the one who had to bring her around, and help her make four or five appointments a day. And they were all over the complex. She would be in a wheelchair, and she is like 150 pounds, plus her leg. And I'd be wheeling her all around the campus."

One of the big surprises for Paulette was learning that, despite her volunteer time with the Reserve and even her high-level connections, she still wasn't fully prepared for the ins and outs of military life as Stefanie recovered.

"Moving into the medical end of it with an injured soldier was a totally different area," Paulette said. "Even though I was familiar with the Reserves I wasn't familiar with the hospital's standard operating procedure. I knew you did things through a chain of command, but the hospital setting was so disorienting because it was a huge hospital and I was just so overwhelmed. And some family members didn't make it there. It was just too overwhelming. The stress of trying to handle the appointments, trying to get appointments, trying to get follow-up care for your soldier, trying to get the right medicine, making sure they're not throwing up, and not leaving them alone because there were suicides going on. You just became so aware of some of these things."

And, of course, it wasn't just Stefanie. All around were visible reminders of the costs of war.

"You would see sights that you would never see," Paulette said. "Someone missing an arm, two arms sometimes. Someone missing all four limbs, missing half a skull. And watching and looking out at how the soldiers were being treated. I thought, 'No, this is not right.' They were treating them like soldiers and they were sick, ill, and injured. At some point the treatment verged on abuse, to threaten them if they missed an appointment? The poor soldiers didn't know. Like my daughter, they had brain injuries. These kids were staying in their rooms. They didn't want to leave. They were depressed, they didn't want to be around people, and no wonder. I just became very involved in her care, and caring about the others."

All this while attending 24-7 to her own child, and sometimes suffering right along with her through what could be grueling physical therapy. As Stefanie's leg healed, with metal plates inside to support her shattered knee, sometimes it had to be manipulated and worked in order to bend the right way, or to ensure maximum movement.

"I could hear her screaming out in the halls when they were doing physical therapy," Paulette said. "She would just scream and cry. They were bending her leg to get it moving. But she was determined that she was going to get it back."

That determination, hours and hours of therapy and care, and a pair of extracurricular activities for the mind and body, paid off. On the physical side, Stefanie was spotted in the pool one day by a coach from the Army's wounded warrior swim team. Stefanie was there for the exercise, and to try to lose weight. But she was encouraged to try out for the Warrior Games, an annual all-forces competition for wounded veterans held at the US Olympic Training Center and Air Force Academy in Colorado Springs, Colorado. Athletes compete in seven sports: archery, cycling, shooting, sitting volleyball, swimming, track and field, and wheelchair basketball. In Stefanie's first year of competition, she won a gold medal in the fifty-meter freestyle and a bronze for the fifty-meter backstroke, and even more in her second year.

"The swimming was so rewarding for me, not just in losing weight but getting me in the mind frame of pushing myself and being able to say, 'Hey, I can do stuff,'" Stefanie said. "The Warrior Games help us focus on our abilities, not our disabilities. It's about what we can do instead of what we can't."

"People couldn't believe how she just blossomed," her mom said. Her twin, who started pushing Stefanie to train for a triathlon, also noticed the difference. In an interview with the *Warrior Transition Command Blog* Jennifer said, "It's great to see her silly, happy-go-lucky personality again. I think her recovery would have taken a lot longer if she didn't have this to work toward."

The idea for further challenging her brain came from Paulette. She had noticed that the computer games Stefanie was given to stimulate her mind often just put her to sleep instead. Then Paulette met composer and musician Arthur Bloom, a Walter Reed volunteer who founded MusiCorps, which connects wounded warriors with musicians who provide private and group music lessons at the hospital. Stefanie loves music, and she had taken violin when she was little, so Paulette suggested she try again.

"I asked Art if he could arrange violin lessons for Stef, and he did that and more," Paulette said. "He got her a donated violin and arranged for a professional from the community to give her lessons twice a week. Stef was really excited; especially when Art told us her teacher would be Mahoko Eguchi, who was with the National Symphony Orchestra in Washington."

Within a few weeks, Stefanie was beginning to make progress. "She had a good year of lessons, and Art and I saw some real improvement," Paulette said. "Her cognitive skills were getting better, and she was using her memory to remember the musical notes. Plus, her fingers and other fine motor skills were becoming coordinated again."

And, fortunately, despite the trying circumstances, Stefanie was able to retain her sense of humor. One day Paulette returned to their room and didn't see her daughter. She called out her name, but there was no answer.

Stefanie was still in a cast. Where could she go? Mindful of the warning from others to never leave their wounded warriors alone for too long, Paulette said she started "freaking out." She went in the bathroom and pulled back the shower curtain. "Boo!" her daughter shouted, followed by "Gotcha." Paulette said, "I went berserk. Here I was thinking one way, and she's . . . she's a character, let me tell you."

Paulette knows that Stefanie's character actually made a difference in someone else's life too. One day while Stefanie was in the gym, she noticed a man who was working out suddenly drop to the ground. "My daughter, who at that time couldn't even bend her leg, hobbled right over to the man and immediately started giving him CPR. It turned out he was a cardiologist at the hospital and he had a heart attack," said Paulette. "Thanks to my daughter's quick response and her care for other people, his life was saved."

Despite progress in some areas, there were setbacks in others. A particularly hard one for the mother-daughter team came when Paulette was issued an ultimatum by her boss. The firm she'd worked for had undergone some management changes after the death of the boss she adored. The new boss called Paulette, who was then on unpaid leave, about six months into her stay at Mologne House. She was told she would have to make a decision: come back to work or stay with her daughter. So the Reserve volunteer who had fought to bridge the gaps between employers and returning service members, and fought for the rights of others, found herself without recourse when she was called up to serve. It was difficult—the first time she'd been out of work since she was sixteen—but ultimately not a decision she had to wrestle with for long.

"Even though I lost my job, I would do it over again," Paulette said. "I really feel that we were blessed that I was able to be there with her. That's the only way she could have made it."

Closer to what was then home, Paulette increasingly saw problems with the military way of doing business. The move from Walter Reed's Mologne House to Bethesda's Building 62, when the former base was shut down, presented a host of challenges, many of which might have been avoided had those in charge spent more time talking to the wounded warriors and their caregivers, according to Paulette. Concerns were raised about the new building having too few accessible entrances, or housing amputees on upper floors—what happens if there's a fire and the elevators are shut down? Paulette took a visiting US senator through their parking garage one day to show how dangerous it was for the wounded warriors.

Other decisions seemed more arbitrary. The cafeteria in Building 62 was shut down for a time, forcing wounded warriors in wheelchairs and on prosthetic limbs to go elsewhere for meals. That decision was reversed after a tipoff to a local TV news station, and the predictably embarrassing coverage. Nonprofits and volunteers, who can make a huge difference in the quality of life for wounded warriors and their family members, were sometimes hassled by officials instead of being welcomed. And though the moms and other family members were critical to the operation and the recovery of their sons and daughters, they often felt they were discouraged from speaking up.

"I don't think some of the military was that used to working with strong women, women who were mothers," Paulette said. "Because we would ask questions. Instead of saying, 'Yes,' we'd ask, 'Why? How come? What are you doing?' And they didn't like that, so they had trouble with us."

That "us" is what helped see her through. As Stefanie prepared to leave the service, Paulette credits the efforts of volunteers, not the military, with helping her through the mountains of paperwork to ensure that her daughter received the correct benefits. (Just one example: the family compiled two pages of errors from Stefanie's initial Army file, which mistakenly listed her as a man and an amputee.)

"It's been a tough three years," Paulette said. "What got me through were the other mothers that I met, the spouses, my religion, and the love I have for my daughter. I wasn't going to let anything happen to her. Sometimes I didn't think I was going to make it. It was so hard. You're thrown into this space with other people, into a situation that wasn't the greatest, and you see all these catastrophic injuries, and your heart goes out to these service members. I just took it very personally, and I cared about every one of them that I met."

What comes next for Paulette isn't clear. She wants to combine her lessons from the last three years with the volunteer work she continues to do for the military. She has gone from ESGR to the Reserve Forces Policy Board, a federal advisory committee that makes recommendations to the secretary of defense on the Reserves, from their strategies and policies, to their capabilities and effectiveness. She also serves on other committees around Washington that affect members of the military, and their families and caregivers.

Paulette would like to organize a group for Silver Star Mothers—the moms of wounded warriors—that would prepare them for the challenges they'll face, while also making their lives easier by integrating the best of the military and nonprofit assistance that's available. It's the kind of information she never heard offered when she was volunteering with the Reserves and certainly could've used in those first days after learning how badly her daughter had been "banged up." It's the type of information she considers vital to helping vets and families handle the realities of military life and develop long-term coping mechanisms in the event of a catastrophic injury.

"I found a memo from my husband, written ten days after her accident," Paulette said. "Somebody had emailed him and said, 'How's Stefanie doing?' And Al wrote, 'Oh, she seems to be in great spirits. She's on the road to recovery.' And I showed him that the other day and said, 'Look at this,' and he said, 'Boy, did I not know what I was talking about.' Ten days."

"We were shocked, and I think that happens to a lot of families," Paulette said. "They have no idea what they're in for, because you're not prepared for it. It's never addressed in the military. . . . I never thought of Stefanie getting injured. I thought either it would be she is going to get killed, or she's going to be back."

Stefanie has medically retired from the military and is working for the court system in Dover, Delaware. She continues to be involved in the Warrior Games, and despite predictions that she would never run again, she's doing exactly that, though it hasn't been easy.

"I tried doing a 5K at the hospital a year before I left," Stefanie said. "I was in so much pain I started crying."

She didn't give up and switched to running on grass to protect her knee. When that went well, she pushed herself even further, signing up for the Army Ten-Miler again, the same race she trained so hard for before her last deployment.

"I trained all summer," Stefanie said, "and wound up coming in only twenty or thirty seconds off my time from before."

What's next for Stefanie, whose mom has set such an example of strength and determination?

"I really want to run a marathon. I want to get that 26.2-mile sticker."

TEN

Derek McConnell and
Siobhan Fuller-McConnell, Esq.

L IKE SO MANY PROUD MOTHERS, SIOBHAN FULLER-MCCONNELL KEPT
track of her son's accomplishments. In one poignant blog post she
listed many of his milestones, including his first smile, his first words,
the first time he rolled over on his own, his first time standing, and, on one
particularly exciting day, his "FIRST STEPS!!!"

But Siobhan was not describing the accomplishments of an infant. Her
son Derek was twenty-two years old when she wrote that blog item on
March 6, 2012.

It had been a little over seven months since then–Private First Class
Derek McConnell had been blown up after stepping on an improvised
explosive device while on patrol in Afghanistan. He lost both of his legs.
His right arm was broken, and the skin torn off, severing nerves, tendons,
and muscle in the process. He had a fractured skull and a fractured pelvis.
His jaw was broken, and several of his teeth were knocked out. There were
blast and burn wounds almost everywhere that he wasn't covered by body
armor, and he suffered internal injuries as well.

"They had twenty-five seconds to get to Derek to save his life, otherwise
he would have bled out," Siobhan said. "That's what they told me later, that
they were on him instantly. He had no vitals when they took him into the

Kandahar hospital. He had no vitals, and they brought him back. So, basically, he died on the battlefield."

From that point every milestone, any milestone, was a miracle. "When Derek came to Walter Reed, he was the soldier no one expected to live," his mom said.

Yet, miraculously, he did. And thus began the milestones. The big smile came at Bethesda, a week after the blast. (His fiancée, Krystina Dressler, had just told him that her mom was going to kick his ass for getting hurt.) His first words were spoken just a few days later. "I'm sorry this happened," he said. Derek wanted to let his family know that he was sorry for what they were going through as a result of his injuries. He also had one simple request: "A chocolate milkshake." (Request denied. His first food came in September, and it was, sadly for Derek, Jell-O.)

In December, Derek rolled over in bed by himself. He stood up for the first time a month after that. Then came the big day. He took his first steps on February 9—207 days after his injury, as Siobhan would dutifully record.

While much of her entry concerned his personal triumphs, Siobhan, who is also an attorney, meticulously noted his many medical firsts: the first day off of the ventilator (for four hours); the first day off of dialysis; the first phantom pain ("This is actually a good thing because it means the nerves woke up," Siobhan recorded); the first day in a wheelchair; first trip back to intensive care unit; first time off "trach." Siobhan created this list a week after Derek did something that some had feared he might never do: spend his first night as an outpatient.

Siobhan also routinely totaled up all of the medical care received to that point: 228 days in the hospital, 36 surgeries, 19 procedures, 129 blood products, countless CT scans and X-rays. ("Too many," she noted. "Basically, he glows, and his kids will be born with three arms.") He had spent 53 days in the ICU, 54 days on a ventilator, 98 days on oxygen, and 114 on contact precautions (people had to wear gowns to enter his room). He was taking 16 different medications when he was discharged, and 34 different medical teams had been involved with his care.

When Siobhan made all of those entries, it had been less than eight months since Derek was wounded, but it seemed a lifetime ago in terms of her perception of the world. "I didn't have a real understanding of what the injuries could be," Siobhan said. "I knew that if I got a knock on the door that was a bad thing. But the whole concept of the injuries—you hear about the Wounded Warrior Project, you see the commercials on TV, so it's sort of out there—but you don't really understand it until you live it or see it."

Siobhan's family has a proud military heritage that can be traced back through several generations. Siobhan's paternal grandmother put together a framed history of her family members who served, both in the United States and abroad. That grandmother's father, a Scot, was a prisoner of war during World War I. Siobhan has the letter, on Buckingham Palace stationery, from King George V to her great-grandfather. One of her grandmother's brothers was killed in World War II, and another was awarded a Bronze Star. Two brothers of her paternal grandfather died in that war. Siobhan's father enlisted after World War II, and he would later share stories of his time in Germany with Derek and his four siblings.

Derek's father, Kevin McConnell, is a Marine veteran of the first Gulf War. He and Siobhan met at the ticker-tape parade in New York City honoring the veterans of that conflict. They were married soon after, each of them bringing a child from a previous marriage. Siobhan had Michael, and Kevin had Derek. They adopted each other's children, and the boys hit it off from the start. "They started to live together when they were three and four years old, and they bonded as brothers and were best friends," Siobhan said. Kevin and Siobhan had three more children together, Sean, and twins Kellina and Ryan. After the couple divorced, Siobhan said the military was often discussed as a career option. "Being the single mother of five children, I couldn't afford five college educations, so growing up we always talked about the military as being a possible way, with the GI Bill, to pay for college," Siobhan said.

Michael went first, enlisting in the Navy after graduating from high school in 2007. He had been pursued by the Marines, and was interested, but Siobhan asked him to at least talk to recruiters from other branches of the service to explore the options. As it turned out, Siobhan said, "He really liked what the Navy had to offer him—jobs, education, and benefits. It's the recruiter's job to sell it and make it amazing. And the Navy recruiter did a better job than the Marines and the Air Force. And what made mama happy was that he wouldn't be on the front line. He'd be safe on a ship—relatively safe."

Derek graduated a year after Michael, and his grades made the military a likely option as well. "Derek got through high school with a smile and his charm," his mom said. "He started the school year off with a backpack, a notebook, and a pen. Just one pen. By the end of the school year, he might've still had the pen. He didn't do his homework. He didn't study for tests. He didn't do much of anything at all. The teachers loved him, and he passed."

His lack of interest paid off in one respect. It led to meeting Krystina. "Derek met his fiancée because he cut class and was hanging out in her classroom to talk to her teacher," Siobhan said. "He would cut his own class and go in and sit and hang out."

After graduation, Derek moved to Virginia for the summer to work in construction with his dad. While there, he started talking to a Marine recruiter. Siobhan warned him that he should give it serious thought before making a decision. "I tried to talk him into the Navy, but he wouldn't let me," Siobhan said. "He was all gung ho. He wanted it. I didn't. I respect the Marines, but I was afraid of him getting hurt, or worse." He signed a delayed-entry contract that eventually fell through when the Marines couldn't guarantee him a spot in the infantry. The Army was more accommodating, and, after his training, Derek was assigned to the 2-87 Infantry Battalion, B Company, at Fort Drum in upstate New York, home of the 10th Mountain Division. They were already preparing for another deployment to Afghanistan when Derek arrived, and would leave on March 18, 2011.

"We had many conversations before he left," Siobhan said. "He was looking forward to it. He felt he was doing something good, that he was protecting our freedom, and ensuring our way of life. He really wanted to serve. He bought into the idea that we were going over there to help the Afghani people get a better way of life. And he wanted to help, he wanted to serve." His mom had misgivings, but said, "I was very proud of him. It takes a lot of courage to knowingly go someplace where people get injured and killed."

Once in Afghanistan, Derek divided his time between a forward operating base (FOB) and command outposts (COPs). "If an FOB is a mobile home, then a COP is a tent in the middle of the wilderness," Siobhan explained. "At the FOB they had access to the Internet, they had Facebook, they had telephones, and they had showers. It was okay living. The COP had none of that. So when he was out at the COP, there was no way to contact anyone."

At the time, Siobhan was practicing family law for a firm in Nutley, New Jersey. While in the office, she'd keep her Facebook page open, hoping for a sign that Derek was online.

"Military moms on Facebook, we wish each other a 'green-dot day,' " Siobhan said, meaning the symbol that indicates when a Facebook user is online. "I would sit in my office, and every five to ten minutes I would click on. I wasn't on Facebook sharing and chatting and all of that. I had it simply on for Derek. When I would see his green dot light up, I would send him a message and we could have a brief conversation. I knew he was okay."

She recalls their conversation on July 22, 2011: "He told me he had to go. He had to get to bed because he was going on patrol early the next morning. I always signed off our conversations with, 'I love you. Be safe.' And the next morning, Saturday morning, 9:28 in the morning, my phone rang. I did not recognize the phone number. I almost didn't answer it. And it was a captain from Fort Drum letting me know that Derek had been blown up."

Siobhan wanted to know if others had been hurt as well. Having met some of the other young men in Derek's unit, she was concerned about them too.

"I met so many of these kids and just loved them," Siobhan said. "So many of them promised to bring Derek home to me in one piece. And, after the accident, they all contacted me, apologizing. This is what weighs on these kids' minds when they get back from war. I didn't blame them, but they blamed themselves."

In fact, someone else had been injured that day. Derek's unit had been called in to secure the landing zone for that soldier's medevac helicopter. As they were leaving the position, working their way through a minefield, Derek stepped on an IED. Fortunately, only the blasting cap went off. It was enough to knock Derek on his rear end, and for his sergeant to tell him how lucky he was. They even took a picture of a laughing Derek holding the dud IED.

"They gave him the opportunity to stand down, and Derek said, 'No,' " Siobhan added. "Two steps later, he stepped on the IED that took him out."

He was immediately medevaced to Bagram Air Base, and then transferred to the US military hospital in Landstuhl, Germany. Siobhan was told that if he missed two transports to the States, or if he took a turn for the worse, she would be flown to Germany. During his time there, while in a medically induced coma, he remained in critical condition. "He was stabilized," Siobhan said, "but it didn't look good."

"That was the hardest thing," Siobhan recalls. "Derek was on the other side of the world, and injured, and I couldn't get to him."

From the time he was injured—to his flight to the United States six days later—the Army was checking in with Siobhan regularly. But the information she received could vary dramatically. "I was told that Derek had lost his arm. I was told the arm was fine. I was told the arm was broken. All the same arm," Siobhan said. "I was told he lost both legs below the knee. I was told that he lost both legs above the knee. I was told that the left leg was fine, but that he lost the right leg below the knee. So I decided that all I want to know is, 'Is he still breathing? Is he still alive?'"

She also called the ICU in Germany, at one point asking that the phone be placed next to Derek's ear so that he could hear her voice. "They say when you're in a coma you can hear what's going on around you," Siobhan said. Through her friendships with other Army moms, a contact was made with a military spouse in Germany, and that woman would visit Derek, talk to him, and report back to Siobhan on what she saw and heard. Another contact, a corpsman at Walter Reed, gave her a heads-up when Derek was finally on a plane home—beating the official channels to the punch. "She said: 'We're getting him. He is definitely on the manifest, and he is flying in tonight,' and that's when we got on the road," Siobhan said. "So when the Army called me to tell me he was coming in, I was pulling in to Bethesda. I was already there."

When the ambulance arrived with three wounded warriors, Siobhan was close by. Derek was the first one off of the vehicle. As soon as he was strapped onto his gurney, a captain signaled to Siobhan. "I ran over, I kissed the top of his head, and they whisked him away," Siobhan said. It was heartbreaking to see how badly injured he was.

Little did she know at the time that he was going to get much, much worse.

"It was horrible seeing him like that," Siobhan said. "He had black eyes, his skin was yellow. But, you know, the SpongeBob look was a lot better than the Barney [the Dinosaur] look that came ten days later. When he turned septic, he blew up and turned purple. He was completely purple."

The force of an IED explosion can drive soil deep into the massive wounds of the injured soldiers and Marines. Though the wounds will later be cleansed, the first priority on the battlefield when limbs are lost is to stop the bleeding, often with tourniquets. Any dirt trapped inside can result in massive infections of the bloodstream. That happened to Derek not long after his arrival at Walter Reed.

"On August 8, he went into full-system shutdown," Siobhan said. "The soil got more embedded into him, and got into his blood, so he went septic."

The family was there in force for Derek from the very first day: Siobhan, Krystina, Michael, who was now home from the Navy, Kellina, Ryan, and Sean. They would take turns going from the ICU to their room, or for a shower or a few hours of sleep, but someone was always with him. If they weren't in the ICU, they were in the day room, waiting for a doctor to arrive. "You never knew when they were going to come through," Siobhan remembered. "I needed to see them and talk to these doctors. I was Derek's medical power of attorney, so I was making all the difficult decisions about his care and what needed to be done."

Derek learned how badly he was injured on August 3. He was off of the ventilator for a few hours and was able to talk, though of course still groggy from the medication. He told them he wasn't sure if he could make it. He kept apologizing. "I never meant for this to happen," Siobhan remembered him saying. But then he asked Krystina to put his feet up. She told him she couldn't. "You can," he insisted. "Put my feet up." They went back and forth, she asking him how, he insisting it could be done, even suggesting she just raise that end of the bed. Krystina and Siobhan kept looking at each other.

Finally, his mom said, "Derek, Krystina can't put your feet up. They're not there."

"Where are they?"

"They're in Afghanistan."

He looked straight at her, "They're where?"

"They left your legs in Afghanistan. The choice was your life or your legs, and they chose your life."

His response? "Fuck it, I'll get new legs."

For a brief moment, just being able to hear his voice, and having Derek be able to finally express himself, Siobhan felt she was getting her son back. But then his lungs failed, and he had to be re-intubated.

Besides keeping notes, Siobhan also took copious pictures of Derek on a daily basis. From that first week, she has one of Krystina by his bedside. They are holding hands, and watching TV. She's wearing a gown, gloves, and a mask. "He was awake, but how much he knew or really understood what was going on we really don't know," Siobhan said. "He was conversing with us, and we were talking back, but he has no memory of any of that."

Siobhan spent evenings curled up in a chair by his bedside, catching a few hours of fitful sleep. When Derek began having nightmares, she would hold his hand, resting her head on the bottom of his bed. "He didn't have legs there, so I could put my head there," she said. She shrugged. "Amputee humor."

Humor helped the family, and Derek, cope. "You have to laugh," Siobhan said. "We had people walk by our room and give us the dirtiest looks because we would be sitting in the ICU laughing. Every single day we found something to laugh about." It was when Derek was first being taken out of his coma that Krystina told him her mother was going to kick his butt. That made him smile. "That was a big deal, that he smiled," Siobhan said. Later, Siobhan would joke with her amputee son about being taller than him again. "Wait," he told her, "I'll be taller than you again soon." And once he had prosthetic legs, he was.

The families of wounded warriors learned how to adapt to such high-stress, unusual situations. "Around Walter Reed, you hear things that you don't hear anywhere else," Siobhan pointed out. "Like, 'Hey, can you get me my legs?' 'Hey, don't knock my leg over.' 'I'm tired. I'm just going to take my legs off.'" There's even a table with a sign: "Stump socks, not hats," warning passersby not to confuse the knitted items that the wounded warriors use on their stumps for caps.

Derek took the initiative to help visitors adapt to this environment and his situation. When his ten-year-old cousin was coming to visit for Thanksgiving, clearly nervous about seeing Derek, whom he idolized, for the first time since the explosion, Derek greeted the boy by ripping off his sheets, wagging his stump and saying, "I ain't got no legs. I ain't got no legs." "He was just laughing about it," Siobhan said. Other times, if a guest was not so welcome, he might "burp" his colostomy bag, and the resulting smell was sure to cut the visit short. One particularly tense day, annoyed with Derek, both Siobhan and Krystina had to step out of the room. From the hall they could hear an apologetic Derek singing at the top of his lungs, "Baby, come back. You can blame it all on me." Siobhan said, "He had all the nurses laughing."

The humor helped, but it didn't change how seriously hurt Derek was. Siobhan said, "For the first two weeks, we heard so much negative, how grave it was, how bad it was, how we didn't know if he was going to survive another twenty-four hours or not, how he was the sickest patient in the hospital." And still it got worse. August 8, the day Derek went septic, changed everything. "The only doctor who ever said things in a positive way sat me down and said, 'I don't know if I can save him,' " Siobhan said. "That crushed us."

Derek hadn't slept the night before, and neither had his mom. He was supposed to receive a tracheostomy the next morning. Still intubated, he couldn't sit up or talk. He would point to the tube down his throat and mouth the word "When?" to his mom. "The night nurse and I were counting down the hours to his surgery," Siobhan said. Derek was also having trouble with his blood pressure, and Siobhan had been warned by the doctor to notify the nurse on duty should his numbers fall below a certain level. They did, and when Siobhan went looking for help, she couldn't find her nurse.

Usually, Siobhan said, nurses let her know if they were stepping away for any reason. That hadn't happened this time. Siobhan found the nurse in charge, and Derek's nurse returned shortly after that. Words between Siobhan and the nurse were exchanged, and the situation remained tense until the arrival of Dr. Obi Ugo, who was handling Derek's surgery. Siobhan remembered, "He says, 'Mom, you need to go get a cup of coffee, relax. He's in my hands now.' "

After the surgery, the doctor was considerably more somber. Siobhan was told that Derek was septic, an infection that could result in his system shutting down. That was when Dr. Ugo told her he didn't know if he could save her son.

On another night when Derek seemed in danger of going septic again, the nurse on duty helped ease Siobhan's anxiety, even though she was again watching his blood pressure numbers drop. "I knew something was wrong," Siobhan said, "but he just was very calm and he said, 'Don't worry. Dr. Ugo will be here soon.' " When the resident arrived, he persuaded Siobhan to leave for the night and rest, and she actually could. "It was okay. It was Dr. Ugo. I knew he was going to do everything he could," Siobhan said. Both Dr. Ugo's calming demeanor, and the evident concern he had for Derek, led Siobhan to trust him as she would few others. "He told me that Derek was the first patient he saw when he came on duty, and the last person he checked on before he left," Siobhan said. "He was also the last patient he thought of before he fell asleep, because Derek was that sick and needed that much care."

Though there were rare exceptions—and those exceptions would lead to Siobhan's "these people can't be around Derek" list, counsel that the hospital actually accepted—Siobhan has high praise for the staff and others at Walter Reed. "I met the most wonderful people at the worst time of my life," she said. "If it hadn't been for them, I wouldn't have gotten through it. When I felt myself losing it, there was always somebody there to talk me down, one of the doctors or nurses that I love, or another mother or a wife, even another amputee." One mother even gave her a bracelet, which Siobhan still wears, because the words on it reminded her of Siobhan: "Friend, mom, caring, cherished, unconditional love, loving, mother, generous, devoted, hero, kind." Words that describe many of the moms at Walter Reed.

It would take four months before the doctors were willing to declare Derek "out of the woods," a metaphor that the main trauma doctor, Philip Perdue, deployed regularly as he charted his patient's progress. He's closer to the edge, he would tell Siobhan. He can see the edge of the woods. Or, we can now see him, but we just can't get him out yet. Or, he's still camping. "For four months, we had a daily fear," Siobhan said. "They couldn't tell me if he was going to live."

They got the word in November. His blood was finally clear; he was breathing on his own. There were still innumerable problems, but he'd made substantial progress.

"It was a very happy day when Dr. Perdue walked into the room and said: 'He is out of the woods. They're in the rearview mirror,' " Siobhan recalled. "Oh, yeah, they heard us cheering down the hall."

He would still spend three more months in the hospital. And though moved from the ICU in September, he had a corpsman in his room 24-7 for about two months. He had pneumonia until November, and returned to the ICU three more times, twice for breathing issues, and once because his potassium level was dangerously high. Siobhan remembers the day of the high potassium level for another reason: she was fired from her job.

It was already a difficult time. Derek was back in the ICU, and also upset because Krystina was going home to New Jersey for the weekend, a first for her. This was two months into Derek's stay at Walter Reed, and would be one of only two times she would leave Washington during the seven months he was an inpatient. At the same time, Siobhan was visited by members of the law firm where she was an associate practicing family law. Initially, when she first left for Walter Reed, she had offered to work from the hospital, or figure some other way to contribute. But she was told not to worry, to concentrate on Derek. "All right," she thought, and told them she hoped to be back in about two weeks. Of course, in the days before Derek arrived from Germany, she really had no idea what she would soon be facing.

"People don't realize what happens when these guys are injured," Siobhan said. "I didn't know what I was walking into. I honestly thought that I would come down, I would be with Derek, I would get him situated, and he'd go off to rehab. He would do his rehabilitation, and I could come visit him on the weekends, or at least every other weekend. . . . I didn't expect him to be so close to death. I didn't expect, as one doctor told me, 'He's knocking on death's door, and it isn't opening yet.' " Once faced with the seriousness of Derek's wounds, work was the furthest thing from her mind. "I didn't know he was that sick," Siobhan said. "What I saw, it was just so overwhelming. Honestly, I wasn't thinking about the job and everything. I was thinking, 'I have to keep this kid breathing. I have to make sure that his medical care is good and that no one makes a fatal mistake.' "

Two months later came the visit from the firm.

"They showed up out of the blue and said: 'We lost our biggest client; there is nothing for you to return to.' They did offer a nice severance package," Siobhan recalled. She understands that it was a business decision, not personal, but adds, "It made my situation a lot harder. I would've liked to have known that I had something to return to, you know, even if they said, 'We're not going to pay you while you're away. When you get back in town, call us.' "

But here's how she describes her reaction to the firm's representatives: "Okay, thanks for coming. I have to get back up to the ICU."

When she returned, she told no one what had happened, but was soon approached by Dr. James West, the neuropsychiatrist who had been working with the family since Derek had arrived at Walter Reed. He told Siobhan that a nurse had said to him, "She's one of the strongest mothers I know, but she seems to be cracking today." Siobhan told him that she lost her job, but insisted that he not tell Derek—at least not yet.

When Derek finally did find out, the sorrow he'd been expressing from the first time he could speak after the blast worsened. "He had a lot of guilt, especially after I lost my job," Siobhan said. "He kept apologizing to me, so we spent a lot of time just talking about how none of this was his fault. He didn't purposefully step on an IED and end up in the hospital to make me lose my job. That's never what he intended. It was just something that happened."

Hours upon hours together drew them closer, sometimes discussing topics that were once too difficult to address, and sometimes with the assistance of Dr. West. "We were able to talk about things we never could before," Siobhan said. "He told me how, when he was a teenager, he resented the fact that I was not his biological mother. He and I were really able to resolve a lot of the teenage angst issues by just finally being able to communicate."

And communicating included joking around with each other. To prepare for getting his prosthetics, Derek was given a "desensitizer." It was a blue sponge on a plastic stick, and he or family members would use it to tap or rub his right stub and left hip (the left leg had been amputated from the hip), making them less sensitive and thus able to endure the use of prosthetics. But it had another application as well. "When Derek would start getting mouthy, we'd start whacking his head. We called the blue sponge the 'Derek beater,' " Siobhan said. Her son would respond by screaming, "Cripple abuse! Cripple abuse!" and calling a "code gray," the hospital signal for security to lock down the ward and remove a disruptive family member or patient. It never worked. Siobhan stayed.

And so did Krystina. If there were discouraging moments at Walter Reed for Siobhan, there was also daily inspiration. And much of that came from her son's fiancée, who gave up her life in New Jersey when Derek was hurt. She not only quit her part-time retail job, but dropped out of the County College of Morris, where she was studying interior design.

"Krystina stayed the whole time," Siobhan said, still in awe. "Nineteen years old. She quit school, she quit her job, and she moved down there. She stayed with me. We actually stayed together. There aren't many young ladies who can live with their [future] mother-in-law for nine months and only get into one argument the entire time. Derek and I had several, but Krystina and I had one." But it was her devotion to Derek that was even more impressive. "She did everything for him," Siobhan said. "She put up with more crap. We saw wives walk out. Oh, yeah, wives who couldn't deal with it, and they left. Not Krystina."

Derek and Krystina weren't officially engaged when she moved to Walter Reed. But they had known each other for four years, and the families were expecting a wedding at some point. Derek had plans to propose during his R&R scheduled for August 2011, one more thing the IED explosion changed.

"She really is amazing," Siobhan said. "The best or worst in people comes out in the most trying circumstances, and that's when you really know the true grit of a person."

Krystina would return to school, changing her major to occupational therapy because of her experiences at Walter Reed. Derek also inspired his sister Kellina, who is studying art therapy, hoping someday to work with autistic children or wounded warriors.

Siobhan's sister, Yvette Maglio, was also a huge help. After first being with their mom in Washington, Kellina, Ryan, and Sean had to return to school in New Jersey, and they moved in with Yvette.

"It was hard on them," Siobhan said. "They had a lot of adjustments to make. Ryan's lung spontaneously collapsed in February, while Derek was still an inpatient. I had two kids in two hospitals in two different states. And Ryan's was life-threatening. The doctor told my sister that if she hadn't gotten him in when she did he wouldn't have made it."

Surprise support also came from Siobhan's congressman, US Representative Rodney Frelinghuysen, who represents New Jersey's eleventh congressional district. He was always accessible, and he or staff members said she could call anytime. They were true to their word—unlike some VIPs who have come through Walter Reed promising support or, in Siobhan's case, jobs. Once, Frelinghuysen showed up at the hospital unannounced because he'd read on Siobhan's blog that she was having a problem. "Anything I need, he's there for me," Siobhan said.

Finally, after seven months, Derek was ready to become an outpatient. He would transfer to an apartment in Building 62 and continue his rehabilitation. He would be allowed one nonmedical attendant (NMA), the person who would help him schedule and keep appointments, ensure that prescriptions were filled and medicine taken, and perform a host of other chores great and small. For some veterans, that role fell to the mom or the spouse. The McConnells planned a different route.

Siobhan said: "I was Derek's nonmedical attendant for the first month, to help him process out, and then Krystina took over from there. I was there to kind of get things situated, so that Krystina knew where she was going and what was happening. Then she took over, and she was great at it."

The three of them moved into Building 62 together for the month of March. In April, Siobhan headed home to New Jersey.

"I had mixed feelings," Siobhan said. "Both Krystina and Derek were very young. And at that point, Derek was taking more control over his care.

I didn't always agree with his decisions, especially that last weekend. I keep saying to myself, 'If only I had been there, maybe he would still be alive.' "

Derek was found dead in his apartment almost one year later, on Monday, March 18, 2013. Krystina tried waking him up for his 7:30 a.m. appointment at the Military Advanced Training Center (MATC), where amputees work out, practice using their prosthetics, and receive occupational and physical therapy. She later wrote: "I tried everything I could think of. I held out hope when I listened for a heartbeat as I tried to wake him and there was none, and even still held out hope when they told me he was gone."

Once Krystina notified the base authorities, she was moved to another apartment. She was allowed to call her mother, so she could come to Walter Reed and be with her daughter. But Krystina couldn't notify Siobhan, who that day was in New York City on a job interview. Army protocol dictates that next of kin be notified in person. Krystina complied with the regulations, until she learned that the Army might not tell Siobhan about her son until the next day. Then she made the call.

"She was hysterical on the phone," Siobhan recalled. "She just kept saying, 'I'm sorry. I'm sorry. I'm sorry.' I said, 'What? Is he in the hospital again? Was he in an accident? What happened? Do I need to come down there?' And then her mother got on the phone. And once I heard her mother's voice, I knew. I knew. So I just sat at the top of the stairs and screamed."

She, Michael, and Yvette drove to Walter Reed that night, and tried to piece together the events leading up to Derek's death.

The Wednesday before, Derek had gone to the emergency room at Walter Reed with severe abdominal pain. Doctors couldn't determine the cause of the pain, Siobhan was told later, but he was admitted, prescribed medications, and released on Saturday. However, for the previous two months, he hadn't been taking any medication, a condition he quite deliberately sought after being on so many drugs nonstop for eighteen months. "He very much wanted to be narcotic-free," Siobhan said. "He didn't like the cloudy feeling. He worked very closely with his doctors, especially his psychiatrist. He called me so excited. He was off all his narcotics. He was feeling great. His head was clear for the first time since the injury. He really felt good."

Siobhan believes that the level of medications prescribed as a result of Derek's ER visit were too much for his then drug-free system to handle.

As she had so often before during Derek's long ordeal, Siobhan, in her grief, turned to her blog:

Dearest Derek,

There are no words. There are no words to describe this feeling. There are no words to describe what is going on in my head. There are no words to explain what happened. There are no words that can make this even slightly better. I can talk and talk and talk but it all comes out in circles, fragments, and empty thoughts. How can I say "good-bye," when I have no words?

The world was a better place with you in it. The people who knew you are better for having you as part of their lives. The world will never be the same. The world is a darker, sadder place now that you are gone.

The emotions, stories, love expressed during our last two days at Walter Reed was overwhelming. The tears shed could fill the Potomac. The laughs as we told our Derek stories still ring through the halls. Everyone who knew you loved you. . . .

What we do know is that you are dancing in Heaven, your body restored. . . . We also know that our lives are irrevocably changed. We went from VA appointments, preparing for retirement, training with an amazing service dog with an angel's name, Gabriel, and planning a wedding, to dealing with Casualty Affairs, muddling through Army protocol, and planning a funeral.

How do we wrap our heads around this? How do I wrap my head around going from a Blue Star Mother, to a Silver Star Mother, to the dreaded Gold Star Mother, all within two years' time?

I could have accepted this better twenty months ago. When you were so sick. When you were in the ICU. When Dr. Ugo took my hand and simply said, "I don't know if I can save him." When Dr. Perdue was in constant touch, giving me his cell phone number, and working so hard to save your life. When I was standing guard at the door, demanding action and refusing to let anyone into the room who did not know you or who would not give exemplary care. I could have accepted it then. Almost.

But now? After twenty months of fighting to get you better? When you were a couple of months from coming home to us?

This is not okay. This will never be okay.

I am angry. I am hurt. I am heartbroken.

Your little lady is the strongest woman I know. She was there for you for the six years since you waltzed into her classroom with a smile, of course cutting your own class to hang out and chat with her teacher. She was there for you for the twenty months you were at Walter Reed. That morning, she was there trying in vain to wake you. But you were gone. You were the love of her life. . . .

I love you. I will always love you. . . .

Rest well, my son, my angel, my hero. You earned your rest.

Stand down, Soldier. Your watch has ended. You are now Heaven Deployed. Never to be forgotten.

In loving memory of my baby boy, my soldier, my hero. Derek Tra McConnell, October 8, 1989–March 18, 2013

ELEVEN

BAND OF MOTHERS

WHEN THEIR SONS AND DAUGHTERS LEAVE FOR BOOT CAMP, MOMS worry about the road ahead. Becoming a soldier or Marine is notoriously grueling work. But the moms also know the training is handled by some of the military's most experienced professionals. When these young recruits head for their first duty stations, they are more than prepared.

But, for the caregiver moms of severely wounded warriors at Walter Reed, there is no training, no way to adequately prepare them for the mission ahead. In order to survive the unthinkable, Stacy, Mary, Lyn, Pam, Carolee, Valence, Tammy, Julie, Paulette, and Siobhan—and countless others—had to learn to lean on each other as a team. From the moment they heard that their sons and daughters had suffered horrific injuries, they reached out for comfort and knowledge from the moms who came before them. They strengthened each other in moments of crisis, adopting their own version of that sacred trust among members of the military: no mom left behind. Though unintended members of an exclusive club, they are now a true band of mothers with a mission of their own: to keep their sons and daughters alive.

As Mary said: "We were thrown together by circumstances that we all wish, hope, and pray that no one will ever have to experience. But as long as there is a war, there will always be a bond between all moms and the military."

To make sure that their children received the best care possible, the Mighty Moms huddled in hallways outside their hospital rooms, worrying about wounds, fevers, and infections. They offered a shoulder to cry on, or a silly joke to relieve the tension. They compared notes on medications, dressing a wound, or cutting through the red tape. They helped each other in other ways too, like providing the names, phone numbers, and emails of the right person to see if they wanted a problem solved ASAP.

"I learned to be resourceful and respectful, but I was a bit demanding about Stefanie's care," Paulette said. "Without those other mothers there, I would never have made it."

One of the best ways to maximize those relationships was by gathering in the early evenings on the "patio" of their living quarters at the old Walter Reed or sitting on rockers near the entrance of Building 62. As the Mighty Moms sat in the wooden chairs, they shared vital information, developed action plans, or just released frustrations. Sometimes it was just the moms, other times the circle grew larger.

Siobhan remembers one evening when her son Derek was rehabilitating in Building 62: "Many nights, we sat outside and chatted, laughed, or played board games. We played Scattergories one night, and when the instructions were to move another player's arms and legs to get others to guess the phrase, a quad amputee yelled out, 'There's only one person on our team with arms and legs. *How* are we going to move them?' We all broke out laughing."

Of course, other times the conversation was much more serious.

"I was one of the activist moms, and because I was on a number of committees both inside and outside of the hospital, and also knew many movers and shakers, I was able to help the other moms quite a bit," said Paulette. "We could see that when we banded together, people really took notice."

One area of concern for Paulette, and many others, was the garage near Building 62, where service members and their families parked, or which they passed through en route to appointments elsewhere on the hospital grounds, particularly in bad weather. "America's Garage," as it is labeled, was more like the Wild West to the moms, a parking free-for-all that lacked clearly marked lanes and adequate speed limits, and was just too dangerous for the wounded warriors, especially those in wheelchairs, to navigate. Asking for improvements through appropriate channels didn't seem to work, so

Paulette took matters into her own hands during a visit from Senator Chris Coons from her home state of Delaware.

"Senator Coons paid a visit to the hospital to see us, and showed up with an entourage of Navy personnel," Paulette recalled. "It was pouring that day, so they arrived in a van, and Stefanie and I met him in the lobby of Building 62." When they had to end the visit in order for Stefanie to attend a physical therapy session, Senator Coons offered them a ride. But, Paulette had another idea.

"I took this opportunity to let them know that we will do it the way we do it every day—walk. Then I immediately extended an invitation to the senator, grabbed his arm, and said, 'Why don't you walk with us?' So, he said, 'Fine,' and we headed toward the garage. During our walk, I let him know about the danger within the garage for our wounded warriors who are amputees and in wheelchairs. I pointed out all the issues about the traffic patterns that were very dangerous. I knew I was in trouble, because I could see that his escorts were annoyed that I whisked the senator away from his entourage, but it was the only way I could talk to him alone."

One week later, Paulette said with a triumphant tone in her voice, "The garage has been retrofitted with large cones and stations throughout that will help keep cars in their designated lanes, and help the wounded warriors and others to navigate the space more safely." Sometimes silence is not so golden.

The Mighty Moms' intervention was also critical in saving the Warrior Café, a full-service cafeteria providing hot meals, fast food, salads, and snacks on the ground floor of Building 62. This popular gathering spot is convenient for the moms and wounded warriors because it is located right in the building where they live, and available to them for breakfast, lunch, and dinner. Too often, after a long day of accompanying their sons and daughters to medical appointments, and tending to their daily needs, the thought of cooking dinner was exhausting. The Warrior Café provided a much-needed respite, and a place where the moms could also socialize and relax.

When word circulated that the café was going to be shut down, the moms were more than furious. "I get it financially," said Julie, "and sometimes there is no one there eating, but still, it is a real lifesaver for the guys and us, too."

The decision meant that, instead of having their meals in the building where they lived, the warriors would "have to walk, wheel, or limp nearly a half mile across the Walter Reed campus to the temporary 'food trailer' for breakfast, lunch, and dinner," as Fox News reported.

A Building 62 Town Hall meeting was held to inform the NMAs and wounded warriors about the changes, but it wasn't to discuss potential options. Residents were told that the decision was a "done deal." But the moms had another more intriguing strategy in mind.

Soon, Jennifer Griffin, the national security correspondent for Fox News Channel, was interviewing caregivers and wounded warriors about the café closing, and her report appeared in August 2013. Julie said, "We were watching the news one night, and the next thing we saw was Carolee on Fox News."

On the televised report, Carolee said: "I was very upset. I felt it was a slap in my son's face as a service member. As many times as he has been deployed—what they were doing to him was a disservice."

Soon after the story aired, officials announced that the Warrior Café would remain open.

"Oh, my God, don't mess with the mothers!" Julie said. "We don't care; we just want to get things done!"

In the emotional, stress-filled life of a caregiver, it was only natural that moms joined forces when it seemed as if the world was against them.

"The medical care at Walter Reed was wonderful, and I can't thank the doctors and all the medical staff enough. They saved Tyler's life," Pam said. "But in terms of helping us, there is no real support here for the moms. They pay us the nonmedical attendant money, but don't really understand what it is like to be here and watch your child suffer every day."

Not every encounter between the moms and the hierarchy escalated to the point where outside help was needed. The Mighty Moms and the military had a similar mission: get the troops well. But their tactics sometimes differed, and each side had to adjust, to a certain extent, to the other. The military was used to a crisp salute and a "Yes, sir" once an order had been issued. The moms don't operate that way. They'll ask "why?" If they think a directive harms their son or daughter, or isn't helping in their recovery; they'll push back. And they won't take "no" for an answer.

"When we first got here three years ago, there were so many people working on our case," Julie recalled. "We had numerous doctors from different disciplines, and even though I was familiar with medical terminology, things could be confusing. We had so many appointments in different buildings, and we had to go all over the base. Plus there was so much paperwork that it was overwhelming."

With so many different specialists working on her son's case, Julie said, it sometimes seemed as if they were competing instead of acting as one team to save Adam.

"The continuity wasn't there," she said. "So we asked for a family meeting, and asked all of Adam's medical teams to be there, too." At one meeting, she suggested some things to make life easier for caregivers. "They did listen to us and, like anywhere, change takes some time, but eventually, they heard what we were saying," Julie said. "If you take control, then things can get done. Things have really changed here for the better."

The team approach, with mom and the medical staff working together, benefited Adam. Doctors wanted to use the Spray-On Skin therapy on him, but needed FDA approval, as it hadn't been used on trauma patients before, just those suffering from severe burns. Thanks to Julie talking to President Obama's aide, and the aide taking action, Adam was able to receive the treatment on a one-use-only basis. Julie took advantage of a presidential visit to secure the okay, and the successful result of Adam's treatment could pave the way for future wounded warriors to receive it as well.

Most often, the Mighty Moms were tirelessly working with each other behind the scenes. Anything that one person learned, whether at Town Hall gatherings or in more private settings, was quickly passed along, and then handed down as new families arrived. They instinctively knew that they needed to help the next mom in line, and never once thought otherwise.

"We would tell each other, and also the moms and wives who were new to the process, what they needed to know when they got here," Paulette said. "Things like being on top of medical appointments, taking charge, and not being afraid, and ultimately, being an advocate for their wounded warrior. We would also help them understand the Med Boards process, how to contact the JAG [Judge Advocate General], and what is a power of attorney. You have to be the one to speak for your child. Otherwise, if left up to a soldier who might be on heavy medication, or not able to understand what is going on, some terrible things could happen. There was never anything we could read on all of these subjects, so the moms had to watch out for everything."

Julie agrees that sharing information is crucial, even lifesaving. "One of the tips I've shared with the other moms is keeping a list of all medications that their wounded warriors are taking. Adam was on so many medications, and I was concerned that, if I weren't there, Adam might not know which ones were which. So I asked the nurse if she could write them down for me. Then I made my own list, and also included the number and the color of each pill, and taped it on the arm rail of Adam's bed. That way, if he wanted to know, he could tell, and eventually, he could monitor them on his own."

Stacy is grateful for the early guidance she received from another mom, and makes it a point to pay that graciousness forward.

"When we first got here, Maureen Crabbe helped me so much," Stacy said. "She counseled me when we were in the ICU, guiding me through the endless paperwork, and helping me understand what to expect. Almost every day we would take long walks around the base, and those walks were lifesavers for me."

Similarly, Stacy was there for Lyn when her son Christian arrived at Walter Reed. Stacy had heard about Christian's injuries from a Marine friend of her daughter-in-law.

"I knew when he was coming to the hospital, and wanted to be there to help his mom," Stacy said. First, she sought counsel from the doctor who had helped her son. "He said that he was not as bad as Mark, so I said to Lyn, 'I want you to know that your son is not as badly injured as my son, and my son lived, so I know Chris will, too.' "

Stacy takes it upon herself to speak to new arrivals. "I am more than happy to do that," she said. "I know this is emotionally taxing for all of the soldiers and Marines who are responsible for taking care of the wounded warriors and notifying their families. One of our friends, Major Richard Burkett, who is a wounded warrior and lives with us in Building 62 with his wife and kids, also visits the families when they first arrive."

Pam reached out to Siobhan, Derek's mom, whom she first met on Facebook, even before she arrived at Walter Reed, in that critical period after learning that Tyler was injured but not knowing if he would live or die.

"I am really not a person who warms up to other people too easily," Pam said. "I keep to myself, in general, but this time I knew I needed help, and thank goodness for the other moms here. From that first time I messaged Siobhan on Facebook, and she put me in touch with another mom, Maureen, who was already at Walter Reed, I knew that the other moms would be my lifeline."

For Pam, who normally is shy and avoids confrontation, learning the ins and outs of the military medical system was a challenge at best. After all, she had some medical training, but not enough to allow her to stay calm when her child was so catastrophically injured. She recalled one piece of advice she received that helped her take charge of Tyler and his care. "I was told early on not to make too many waves," Pam said. "There is a lot of bureaucracy, and the other moms said to just 'go with the flow.' I am not that assertive, but I have seen that you do need to speak up, but do it in a nice way."

Just having the other moms there when needed could make all the difference.

"The truth is I never did really know that this life existed, and the thought of Tyler being injured never crossed my mind," Pam said. "Many of the other moms said the same thing, and it was good to be able to share my feelings and hear their stories as well."

Mary said the moms have become each other's soul mates, psychologists, and girlfriends.

"You need each other for so many things, simple things like taking walks or having a drink," she said. "It's just nice to breathe with people who are our own best support systems. When Stacy wants to go to Costco, I am there, and at least we are getting away for a while. As women, we rely on each other. Women let it out. Men hold it in. Ultimately, we support one another and are each other's sanity."

"There were so many times we helped each other, but sometimes we just dropped everything and sat around and laughed," said Mary. "We would ask each other silly stuff like, 'What did you bring with you to sleep in?' or, 'Why did you pack footie pajamas when your son has no legs or feet?' Even when we laugh, we get strength from each other because we understand."

Their collective strength is also a source of comfort for others at Walter Reed.

Tammy recalls one night when she couldn't sleep, and she headed to the patio about 2:00 a.m. for a cigarette. A young wounded warrior was already out there. He couldn't sleep either. He and his wife were constantly fighting, he told Tammy. He was worried about losing his car and all his money. "I don't know what to do," he told her.

Tammy listened, and then reminded him that he wasn't alone, that there were people who could help. She urged him to seek legal advice at JAG. "Everything you said to me, tell them," she advised. When she saw him a few days later, he thanked her. The couple did divorce, but JAG protected him as much as they could, Tammy said.

Similarly, the moms protect each other as much as they can, whether they are close at hand or far away.

Periodically, wounded warriors' cases are reassessed, and the military will sometimes determine that a nonmedical attendant is no longer needed. The wounded warrior continues with his or her care, but the mom goes home. That happened to Ramona Wasylenko, whose son, Mark, suffered from a traumatic brain injury as a result of a military training accident. Though she'd left the fold, her family of moms always kept in touch.

"They decided she didn't need to be there, so we would check up on her, and we would know if she needed us," Paulette said. "I would call her or message her on Facebook and ask, 'You don't sound right. Do you need help?' You want to help, but not pry."

When Valence learned that Ramona was having a problem with her son, the moms sprang into action. Facebook messages flew back and forth, and the moms tried to figure out how best to get Ramona the support she needed.

"We love Ramona, and Paulette and I talked about what we could do to help," Valence said. "I offered to drive to Boston to be with her, and we all told her that we are there for her. Just say the word and we will all be there." The moms were already making arrangements to ensure the care of their own wounded warriors in case they needed to travel en masse to Massachusetts.

Paulette reached out to Jack Hammond, a retired Army brigadier general who was the executive director of the Red Sox Foundation. "Jack, this mother of a wounded warrior needs help," she told him. He had someone on the phone to Ramona that day. Valence said Ramona was moved to tears at the show of support. She wrote on Facebook, "Just when you think you are going to lose your mind, true angels fly into your life. Thank you, my friends. You have let me rant and you have understood."

After two years of nonstop care for her son Christian, Lyn was also asked to leave Walter Reed.

"I tried to explain that Chris was still in a very fragile and emotional state, and that he still had PTSD, and suffered from depression. He needed me to be with him until he was able to survive on his own," said Lyn. "There is no one else in the world that can care for him like me, and I am fearful that if I'm not there, he will become another tragic statistic."

Lyn turned to Stacy and Mary for advice. After several strategy sessions, they came up with a plan. Lyn would make her case in writing, outlining in detail what she did daily for Christian and why that care needed to continue. "Stacy and Mary helped me outline a document that gave specific examples of what I did for Chris on a daily basis, and also gave me the confidence to present that plan in a professional manner," said Lyn.

The two-page document had more than twenty-three items listed, including: "provide emotional support for his depression, traumatic brain injury, and post-traumatic stress; keep an eye out for dangerous behavior; help him dress into regular clothing and get his prosthetics on; clean the bathroom and shower stall; cook meals and shop for food; plan and administer medications; maintain breathing machine; coordinate medical appointments; manage money; reach things in the cabinets, pantry, and the freezer; and support him when memory and other issues arise."

The day before Lyn's presentation, she rehearsed it in front of Stacy, Mary, and her other Mighty Mom advisors, and they in turn gave her the kind of pep talk that only another mom in her situation could. "Stacy really helped me get mentally tough and make my case in a forceful and strong way," Lyn said. That's clear from the moving words that ended her presentation:

> "Chris still needs me to be with him full-time, until the time comes when he can function on his own. He is my son, and there is no greater love than that between a mother and her child. I hope you will allow me to stay with Chris until he is able to live independently. I am more than happy to work with you on a treatment plan that will make that a reality. Thank you for listening."

To her surprise, Lyn's stay as an NMA was extended until Christian is medically retired. She was very proud of her newfound assertiveness, which she credits Stacy and Mary with helping her discover, and is thankful the military extended her caretaker role.

Like all families, the Mighty Moms spend holidays together, and Stacy had a pre-Thanksgiving gathering planned for caregivers, warriors, and others. However, the day before the dinner, Mark developed a fever and cellulitis and had to be taken to the emergency room. The moms decided to take charge.

The dinner would go on, but Stacy wouldn't have to lift a finger. Lyn whipped up pecan and pumpkin pies, a sweet potato casserole, and other goodies; Mary baked rolls; and the other moms chipped in as well. Stacy wasn't allowed to serve or clean up. She was told to focus on Mark, not her guests. She did, but of course she was thinking of others too. Stacy packed up some food for Mark, but also brought dinner for Julie and Adam, who were still in the hospital. Stacy spent the rest of the evening in Mark's hospital room, along with her daughter, son-in-law, and her grandchildren. While Mark was feeling weak from the infection, when his mom and some friends delivered the home-cooked meal, the relief on his face was hard to miss.

Mary believes that the moms will always stay connected, even long after they leave Walter Reed. "Over time, we have bonded with each other so much," she said, "and I hope those bonds will last a lifetime. Yes, our lives have taken a 180, and all of our plans have to be rewritten, but we are survivors and strong. You can take on anyone or anything as long as you are united. That is why all of us have this strong bond."

Stacy often says how much she misses the moms and their soldiers and Marines when they leave Walter Reed, and loves them as much as her own son. "You get so attached to the other moms and also their kids," Stacy said. "I miss them so much when they are gone because we are just like family. Their kids are our kids, too."

Helping to ease the pain of these inevitable separations are the "See Ya Later" parties sponsored by Luke's Wings and the Freedom Alliance, Colonel Oliver North's foundation. As each mom and her wounded warrior prepare to leave Walter Reed, they are the guests of honor in an emotional tribute to their courage, sacrifice, and heroism.

Pam speaks for many of the other Mighty Moms when she says, "I couldn't have made it at Walter Reed without the other moms. We all learn through each other's experiences, and they always pass along their experiences, and for that I am so grateful. If we don't have the other moms, we don't have anybody."

TWELVE

FAVORITE MIGHTY MOMS' CHARITIES

I T TAKES A NATION TO REPAY THE DEBT OWED TO WOUNDED WARRIORS.
While each of the Mighty Moms hopes that her son or daughter will
be able to live as independently as possible, she also knows the realities
of the road ahead. Regardless of the level of self-sufficiency each wounded
warrior attains, the support he or she will need in the future is endless.

While their medical care is provided by Veterans Affairs for life, the costs
of everyday living are astronomical. Homes need to be built that can accommodate the needs of amputees and those suffering from traumatic brain
injuries. Families will need to purchase land where those "smart homes" can
be built. They will need specialized vans to carry their wheelchairs, and different types of wheelchairs that they can use indoors or outside. Some will
need assistance getting to and from medical appointments, and there will be
travel expenses for specialized care. Parents will either move closer to their
wounded warriors, or face expenses for visits.

Fortunately, there are thousands of volunteers and hundreds of nonprofits ready, willing, and able to fill in the gaps. And many of them have
been doing just that for the Mighty Moms from day one.

Julie credits the Yellow Ribbon Fund, whose mission is to keep families
together during the recovery period, for organizing outings off base for
the moms, which give them time for themselves away from their children's
injuries. She now volunteers for the group. "When you need them, they are
there," Julie said. And she is proud of her daughter for creating a nonprofit

181

of her own, called Wounded Veteran Run, which she started because of her brother, Adam. Julie also is fond of Warrior Events, which she calls a "great organization," and she has high praise for its founders Bob Saunders and John O'Leary from Annapolis.

Stacy is grateful to the Semper Fi Fund for helping with so many of Mark's needs, as well as individuals like Bill O'Reilly, the Fox News Channel host who raised money for specialized track chairs for the wounded warriors—each with a price tag of around $15,000. Also, without Luke's Wings, the moms wouldn't have been able to fly themselves or their family members back and forth to Washington.

Mark, Stacy, Amanda, and Kelly were also special guests of the Tug McGraw Foundation, which treated the family to a backstage concert experience when country superstar Tim McGraw (Tug McGraw's son) was appearing in Washington, DC, along with Kenny Chesney. Mark attended a VIP event before the concert, watched part of the show from the stage, and met Tim in person. He was also invited to attend another concert a year later, but couldn't go because he was in the ER with an infection.

"My, if I couldn't find something good in all of this it would be a shame," said Stacy. "The goodness of people is remarkable, and there are so many who have helped us. In our own hometown, one local company agreed to build Mark a completely accessible garage, and they did it all for free. Then Luke's Wings paid for all of Mark's plane tickets, and had them upgraded to first class to accommodate his wheelchair."

She added, "Semper Fi is always there for you all the time. They will help you because you are not working, help with hotel rooms, flights, rental cars, track chairs, and so much more. They even help us with adaptations of our houses along with the Home Depot Foundation."

Mary also credits Semper Fi Fund, along with the Wounded Heroes Fund, the Cowboy Mounted Shooters, and people at home in Bakersfield, California, for helping Josh and her. "I don't know where we would have been without all of their support and assistance," she said.

Tammy points to Operation Second Chance as making a huge difference, providing support when the military delayed the payments she was due as a nonmedical attendant. "I was broke and didn't want to take money from my household," she said. After the bureaucratic runaround, it was comforting to know that others would help. Similarly, Carolee's family received assistance from the Families of the Wounded Fund, which allowed them to take care of some bills back in Juneau while Tom was an inpatient in Richmond.

"You really need all that support," Julie said. "We are all on a tight budget here. We have lost our jobs and there is a great financial strain, so we really do need the help from all the different organizations."

The Aleethia Foundation hosts weekly off-base dinners for warriors and their families. And Truckin' 4 Troops offers monthly barbecues right on the Walter Reed campus during the summer. All of the Mighty Moms especially appreciate Scott Mallary, the founder of Truckin' 4 Troops, who started his family-run nonprofit by driving to the airport, finding service members returning from combat, and driving them wherever they needed to go for free. Today, he helps the Mighty Moms and their sons with so much more, and has become like a family member to them over the years, hosting barbecues and get-togethers at his home.

Valence said she often looked forward to the respite offered by Aleethia's Friday night get-togethers. "Hal Koster, who is the founder of Aleethia, is a true friend," said Valence, who added that Hal often calls her and Robert to see how they're doing. "Hal was always there for us and still is. I sometimes joke with my husband that me and Hal have a thing going. He means that much to our entire family, and the other families of wounded warriors."

MusiCorps is high on Paulette and Stacy's list of organizations. Founder Arthur Bloom enlisted a musician from the National Symphony Orchestra to give Stefanie violin lessons, which her mom credits with restoring some of her cognitive functions. "Art Bloom is one of the most generous people I have ever met," Paulette said. MusiCorps is giving Mark lessons on the ukulele. Bloom also founded the Wounded Warrior Band, featuring lead singer and double amputee Timothy William Donley. Timothy and the band have played at the Grand Ole Opry and Carnegie Hall and have performed with Yo-Yo Ma, John Waters, John Mayer, and many other famous artists. (Timothy is also now dating Mark's sister, Kelly.)

Another favorite of Paulette's is Operation Homefront, which provides transitional housing for families and wounded warriors who are no longer outpatients but still need access to Walter Reed or other services in the DC area. "When Stefanie retired, she had the option of going back home, but learned about Operation Homefront through a family readiness assistant who worked with the Army Wounded Warrior Program," Paulette said. "We

thought it would be better for Stefanie to live in an apartment in Gaithersburg so she could finish her therapy. They were amazing. They paid for a
great apartment for a year, and all I had to pay for was the food. It gave us
time to transition, so you don't abruptly have to come back to your old life,
and it gives you a chance to come down from all of the stress."

The same group came to Pam's rescue when Tyler was told he'd have
to leave Building 62 because his service dog, Apollo, wasn't certified. "Tyler
just loved that dog, and I couldn't bear the thought of having to separate
them," Pam said. "I got in touch with Operation Homefront and Felecia
Suluki was just wonderful. She was gracious enough to step right in, and also
helped calm me down. She got us in an Operation Homefront apartment
right away."

Warrior Canine Connection, which helps veterans with psychological
injuries train service dogs for other veterans, has a special place in Siobhan's
heart. She met them on one of Derek's worst days at Walter Reed, when
doctors were fighting his blood infection.

"When he was taken off to surgery, Krystina and I left to go get coffee
at Dunkin' Donuts, and we saw the dogs. They were across the room and
I commented to Krystina, 'Oh, look, aren't they cute?' One of them heard
me, and made a beeline for me. She herded me into a chair and then just
leaned against my legs for me to pet her. She's very empathetic. She seems
to know where she is needed, and she will go to that person and just snuggle
in to be petted."

After that, Siobhan made a point of keeping treats in her purse for
when the dogs visited Derek's room, and she is pleased that the organization
has since named one of its pups after her son. "Puppy Derek is a little black
Lab with attitude," she said. "He really embodies a lot of his namesake. He
won't smile for pictures, and he's a brat."

Many wounded warriors have received, or are waiting for, "smart
homes" that are being custom-built for them by the Gary Sinise Foundation
and the Tunnel to Towers Foundation.

"We take for granted all of the little things in life that to us seem simple
but for people like Chris are monumental tasks," said Lyn. "Like reaching
for a glass, or going up and down steps. Knowing that Chris can live in a
home that gives him this kind of independence is a blessing."

Lyn will never forget all that actor Gary Sinise has done for her and her
family. Gary is a regular at Walter Reed, often visiting under the radar. He's
considered the "real deal" among veterans and their families, someone who

is there for them, not for just a photo-op. "He genuinely cares, and everyone here knows that," Lyn said.

To help raise money for the smart homes for wounded warriors, Gary Sinise performs concerts with his Lieutenant Dan Band—named for his character in the movie *Forrest Gump*—in the warriors' hometowns. He and his band donate their time, with all proceeds going toward the construction of the home. And he stays in touch with the families through the process, right up until the warrior moves in.

When it came time for the concert for Christian's home, Lyn was nervous. Her entire family was there, and so were many of Christian's friends, both military and civilian. The outpouring of support from the community was huge. As Christian came up the escalator, wearing his "shortie" prosthetic legs, the crowd roared. Lyn was speechless, her big brown eyes filling up with tears.

She was so proud, watching her son feel the love of the many people who wanted to be there to honor his service and sacrifice. But the day wasn't over. When Gary called Lyn, Christian, and their family up to the stage, her heart was racing. As he sang, she watched him look at Christian with such compassion and caring. She was overcome with emotion, and Christian was feeling the love too. This tough Marine had a hard time holding back his tears. "This was literally the best day in my life—ever," Lyn said emphatically.

The Mighty Moms have provided a short list of some of the nonprofits that have made a difference in their lives:

Adopt-a-Soldier Platoon (adoptasoldierplatoon.org)

Aleethia Foundation (aleethia.org)

America's Fund (americasfund.org)

Armed Forces Foundation (armedforcesfoundation.org)

Blue Star Families (bluestarfam.org)

Combat Soldiers Recovery Fund (combatsoldiersrecoveryfund.org)

Elizabeth Dole Foundation (elizabethdolefoundation.org)

Families of the Wounded Fund (familiesofthewoundedfund.org)

Family and Friends for Freedom Fund (injuredmarinesfund.org)

Fisher House Foundation (fisherhouse.org)

Freedom Alliance (freedomalliance.org)

Gary Sinise Foundation (garysinisefoundation.org)

Help Our Military Heroes (helpourmilitaryheroes.org)

Hero Miles (fisherhouse.org/programs/hero-miles)

Hope for the Warriors (hopeforthewarriors.org)
Luke's Wings (lukeswings.org)
Maryland Patriot Guard (mdpatriotguard.org)
MusiCorps (musicorps.net)
National Military Family Association (militaryfamily.org)
Operation Homefront (www.operationhomefront.net)
Operation Open Arms (operationopenarms.org)
Operation Second Chance (operationsecondchance.org)
Semper Fi Fund (semperfifund.org)
Truckin' 4 Troops (truckin4troops.com)
Tunnel to Towers Foundation (tunnel2towers.org)
USO (uso.org)
Warrior Canine Connection (warriorcanineconnection.org)
Wounded Veteran Run (woundedveteranrun.org)
Wounded Warrior Project (woundedwarriorproject.org)
Yellow Ribbon Fund (yellowribbonfund.org)

•

The Mighty Moms of Walter Reed embrace life's challenges with grace, dignity, determination, compassion, and humor. They, like their wounded warrior sons and daughter, know that sacrifice is at the heart of what matters most. Their love for their children, and their pride in them for risking their lives for our freedom, is evident in everything they do. That is why they are Mighty Moms.

As they move on with their lives, their wounded warriors never far from sight, they know there will be other Mighty Moms following in their footsteps. The experienced caregivers will always be there for the new ones, and for their brave young warriors. Their bonds are unbreakable, their compassion boundless.

It's important that the nation remember their service, as well as those who still serve. As President Bush said in his foreword:

"Tonight, when you go to sleep, remember that at this moment there is a young man and woman halfway around the world, sitting alone in the dark, waiting to go out on patrol. They may be tired, and even a little scared, but every day they put on that uniform and they lay their lives on the line for each of us, and for the United States of America. Say a prayer that they come home safe and sound."

ABOUT THE AUTHORS

Dava Guerin

D AVA GUERIN IS A WASHINGTON, DC–BASED COMMUNICATIONS CON-
sultant and writer and is the communications director for the US
Association of Former Members of Congress in Washington, DC.
She was formerly president of Guerin Public Relations, Inc., a full-service
communications firm, and profile editor of *Local Living Magazine* and *Bucks
Living Magazine*. She worked in senior-level positions for Ketchum public
relations and the Philadelphia Convention and Visitors Bureau. She also
volunteers her time helping wounded warriors and their families at Walter
Reed.

With more than twenty years in the marketing communications and
public relations fields, she has worked with numerous US presidents, including George H. W. Bush, George W. Bush, and Jimmy Carter, as well as President Hamid Karzai and Nelson Mandela. She has also managed visits for
numerous dignitaries and entertainers, including Bob Hope, Sir Elton John,
Tim McGraw and Faith Hill, Lauren Bacall, and many others. She continues
to work with former First Lady Barbara Bush—helping her relaunch her
popular ABC Radio Network show called *Mrs. Bush's Story Time*.

Guerin has also managed national and international public relations programs for many Fortune 500 companies and other organizations, including:
H. J. Heinz; GlaxoSmithKline; the Philadelphia Eagles; Dietz & Watson; US
Health Care; Rohm and Haas Company; Campbell's Soup Company; Man-
nington Floors; and Comcast Corporation, among others.

She also provided media credentialing for more than two thousand reporters who attended the Presidents' Summit for America's Future, which was held in Philadelphia in April 1997, and she was the editor of the 2000 Republican National Convention's *Official Delegate and Media Guide*, as well as one of the chairs of Philadelphia 2000's Marketing to the Media committee.

Guerin has extensive experience in media relations, community relations, special events, and crisis management—from coordinating network live remotes for *Good Morning America*, *Today*, and *Nightly Business Report* to managing international media relations programs for the City of Philadelphia's We the People 200 celebration in 1987, and numerous festivals commemorating the Fourth of July in Philadelphia, such as Welcome America and The Photo of the Century; Live 8; and the Congressional Medal of Honor Society's National Patriot's Award.

Guerin has also managed numerous client crisis situations, including a mass murder, a national brain cancer scare, union strikes, product recalls, and product tampering.

She graduated summa cum laude with an MEd degree in organizational behavior from Temple University, and graduated from Goddard College with a bachelor of arts degree in English and literature. Guerin also attended Rutgers University, and the University of London's summer program focusing on history and literature.

Guerin has provided pro bono services to numerous nonprofit organizations across the country, including the National Archives; was past president of American Women in Radio and Television's Philadelphia Chapter; and is currently on the advisory board of the Tug McGraw Foundation.

Kevin Ferris

Kevin Ferris has been a member of the *Philadelphia Inquirer*'s editorial board since 1995. He currently oversees the Commentary and Sunday Currents sections, and for many years wrote a nationally syndicated column on state and national politics, international affairs, defense, and veterans' issues. His freelance work has appeared in the *Weekly Standard*, the *Wall Street Journal*, and the *Christian Science Monitor*.

Kevin holds a master's degree in international relations from American University in Washington, DC, and a bachelor's degree in mass communications from Virginia Commonwealth University in Richmond, Virginia. He served in the US Army from 1976 to 1979.

Kevin lives in West Chester, Pennsylvania, and has two children.

President George H. W. Bush

George H. W. Bush was sworn in as president of the United States in January 1989 and served until January 1993. During his term in office, the Cold War ended; the threat of nuclear war was drastically reduced; the Soviet Union ceased to exist, replaced by a democratic Russia with the Baltic states becoming free; the Berlin Wall fell and Germany was reunified with Eastern Europe; and he put together an unprecedented coalition of thirty-two nations to liberate Kuwait. He served in the US Navy from 1942 to 1945, and has supported our nation's service members and their families throughout his life. As a champion of public service, he has encouraged all Americans to serve through his Points of Light Foundation, as well as his personal philanthropic efforts. He resides in Houston, Texas, with his wife, Barbara, and their two dogs.

Connie Morella

Connie Morella represented Maryland's eighth congressional district in the House of Representatives from 1987 to 2003, served as ambassador to the Organization for Economic Cooperation and Development from 2003 to 2007, and is now president of the US Association of Former Members of Congress. Already a mother of three, Morella adopted her sister's six children after she passed away from cancer. In her role as president of the US Association of Former Members of Congress, Morella has been a champion of US wounded warriors and has supported them through her organization's charity golf tournament and Salute to Service: Statesmanship Awards Dinner, as well as many other initiatives. She resides in Bethesda, Maryland.